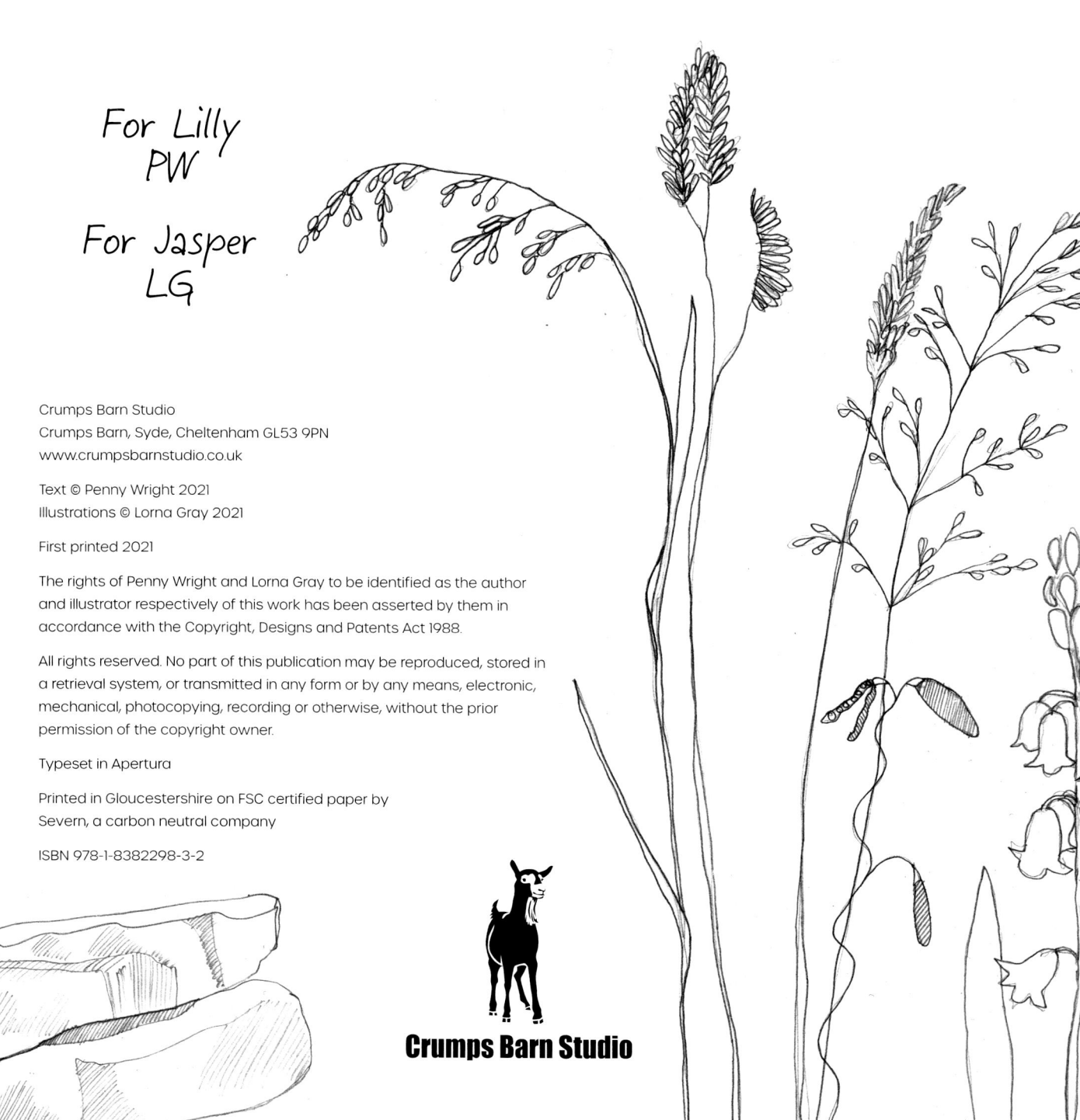

For Lilly
PW

For Jasper
LG

Crumps Barn Studio
Crumps Barn, Syde, Cheltenham GL53 9PN
www.crumpsbarnstudio.co.uk

Text © Penny Wright 2021
Illustrations © Lorna Gray 2021

First printed 2021

The rights of Penny Wright and Lorna Gray to be identified as the author and illustrator respectively of this work has been asserted by them in accordance with the Copyright, Designs and Patents Act 1988.

All rights reserved. No part of this publication may be reproduced, stored in a retrieval system, or transmitted in any form or by any means, electronic, mechanical, photocopying, recording or otherwise, without the prior permission of the copyright owner.

Typeset in Apertura

Printed in Gloucestershire on FSC certified paper by Severn, a carbon neutral company

ISBN 978-1-8382298-3-2

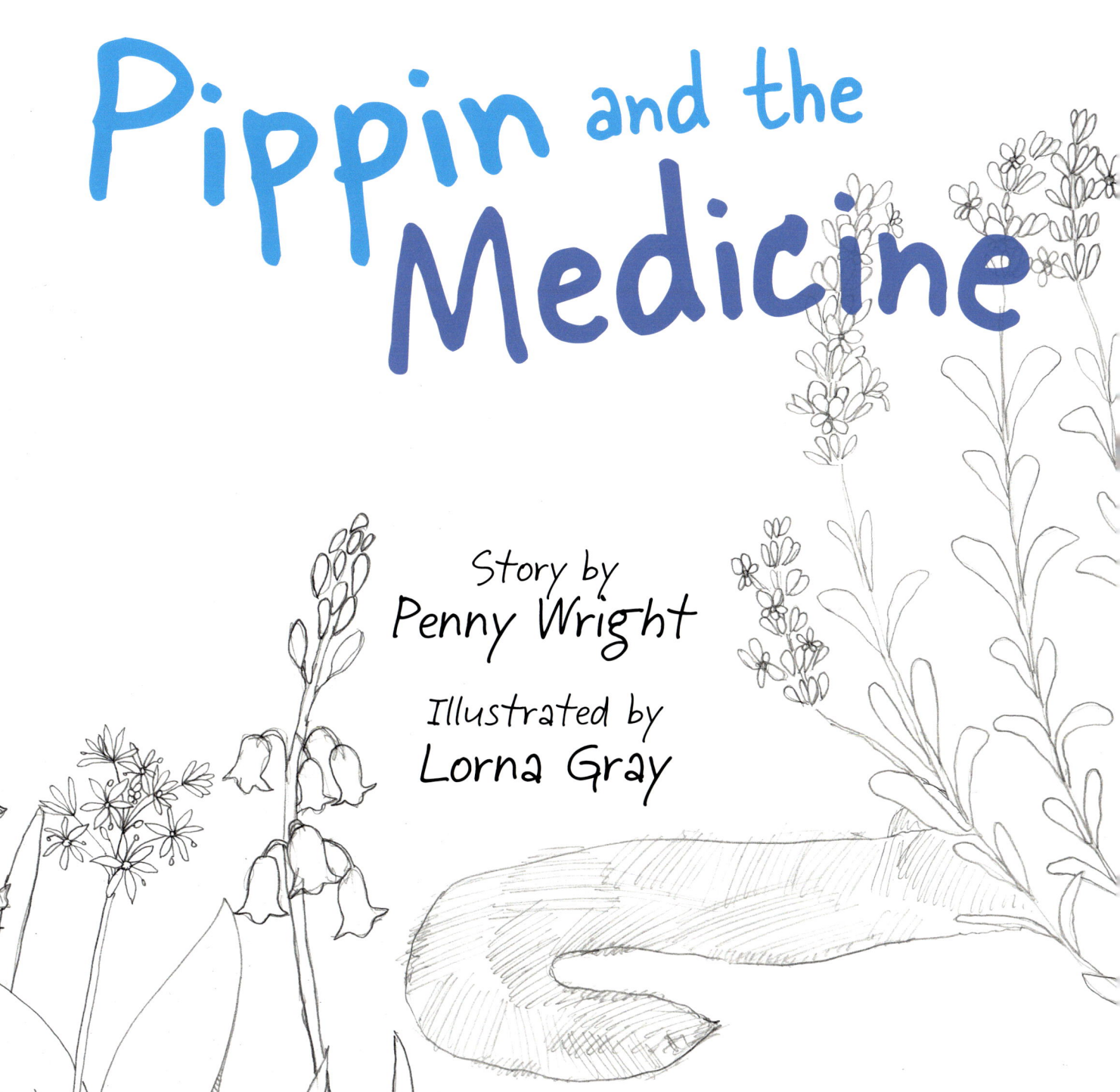

Pippin and the Medicine

Story by
Penny Wright

Illustrated by
Lorna Gray

Once upon a time there was a little black and white cat called Pippin.

Pippin was very cute and a bit daffy.

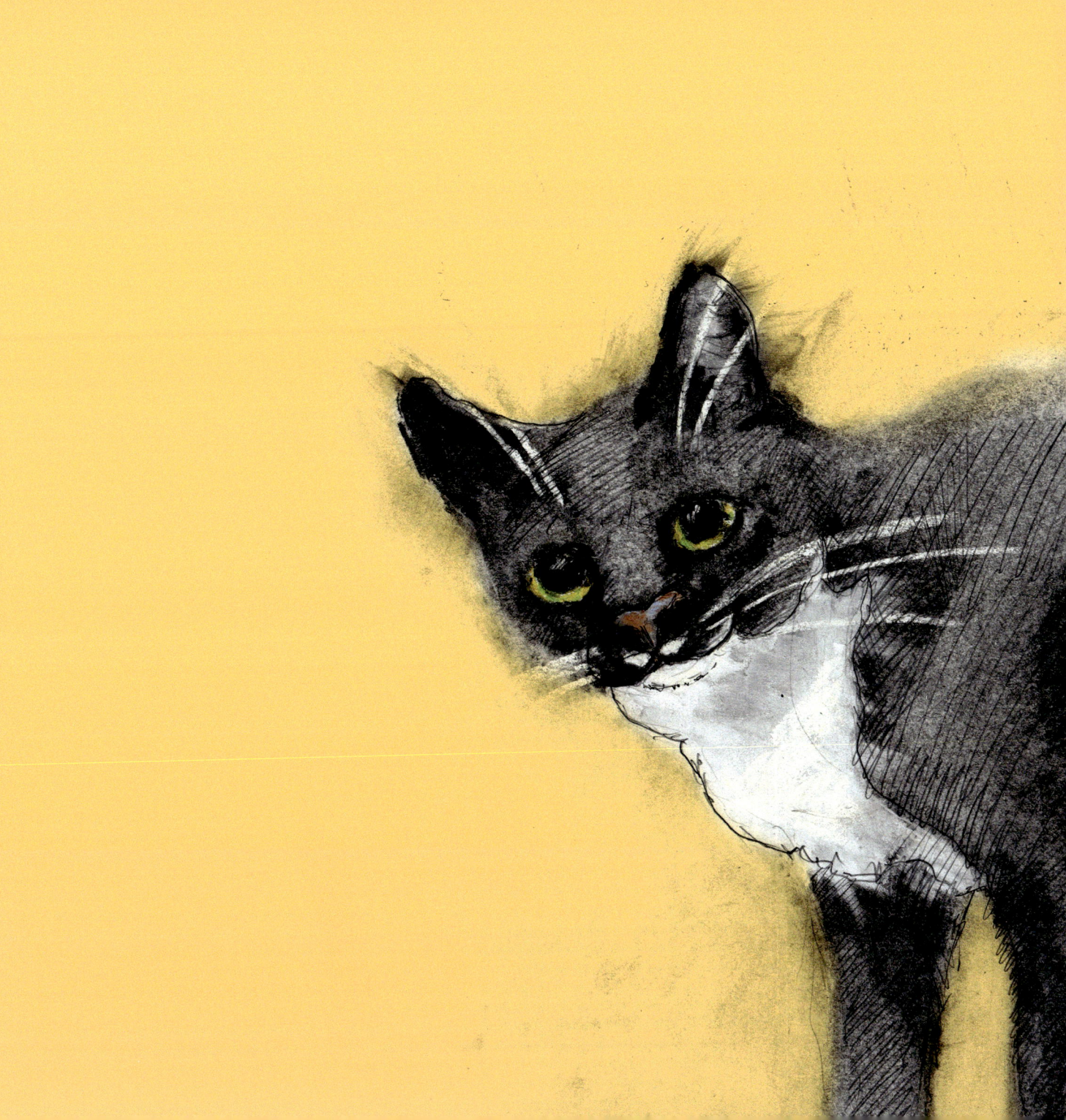

He had white socks and a white shirt.

He had a black coat that was too small for him and did not meet in the middle.

He had white whiskers and amazing white eyebrows.

He had a very soft bit just behind his ears.

And he had very bad table manners.

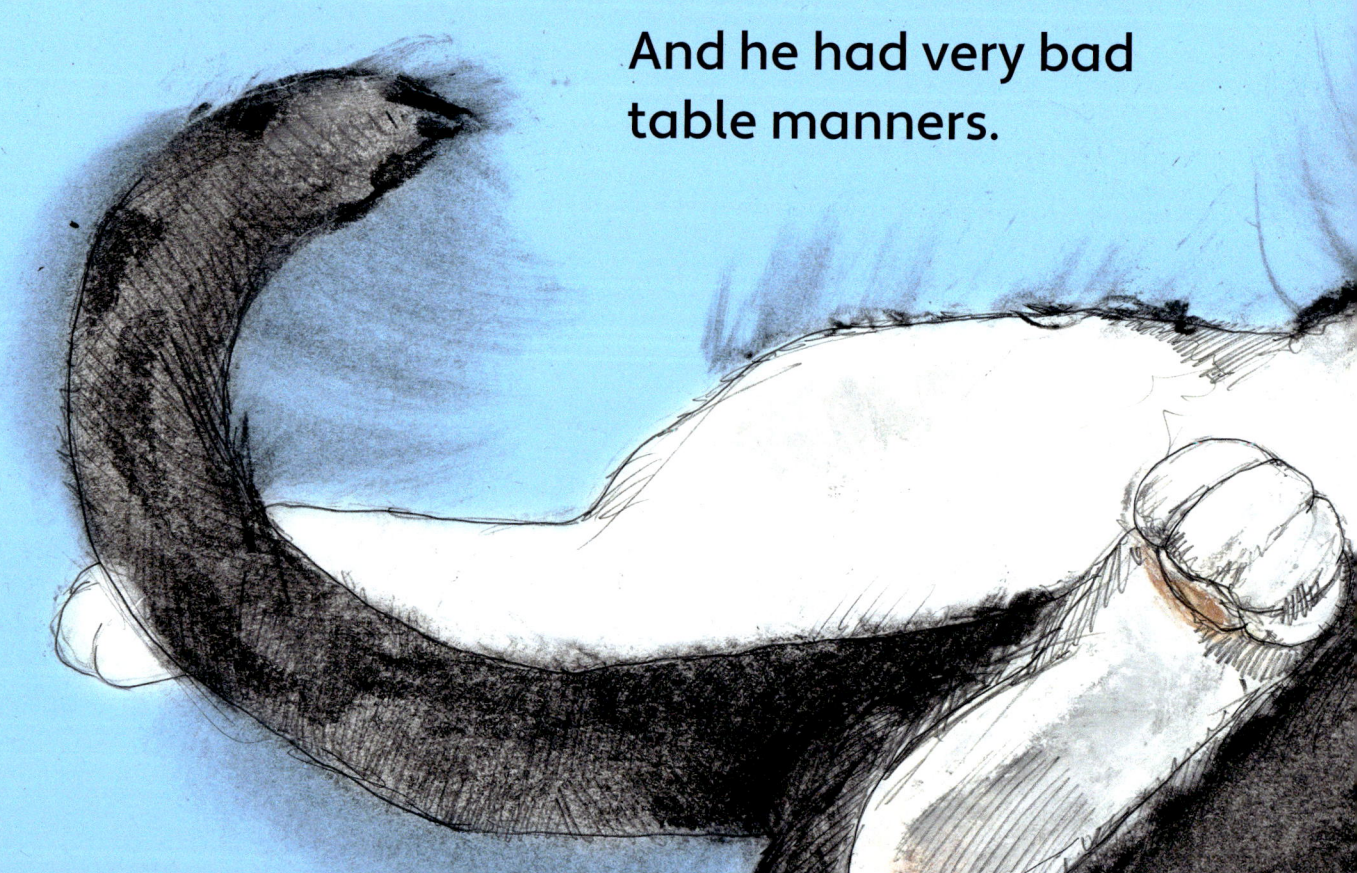

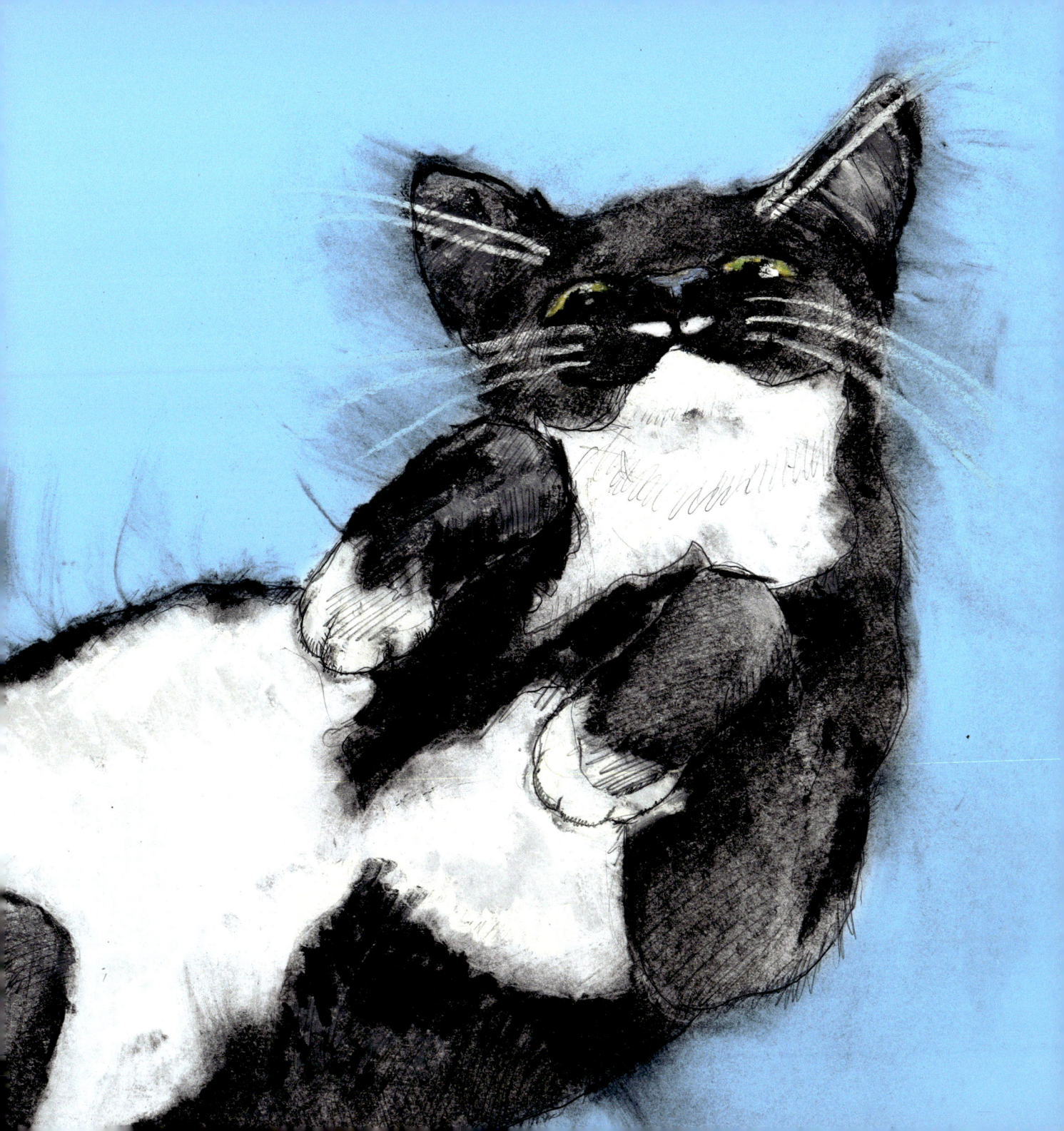

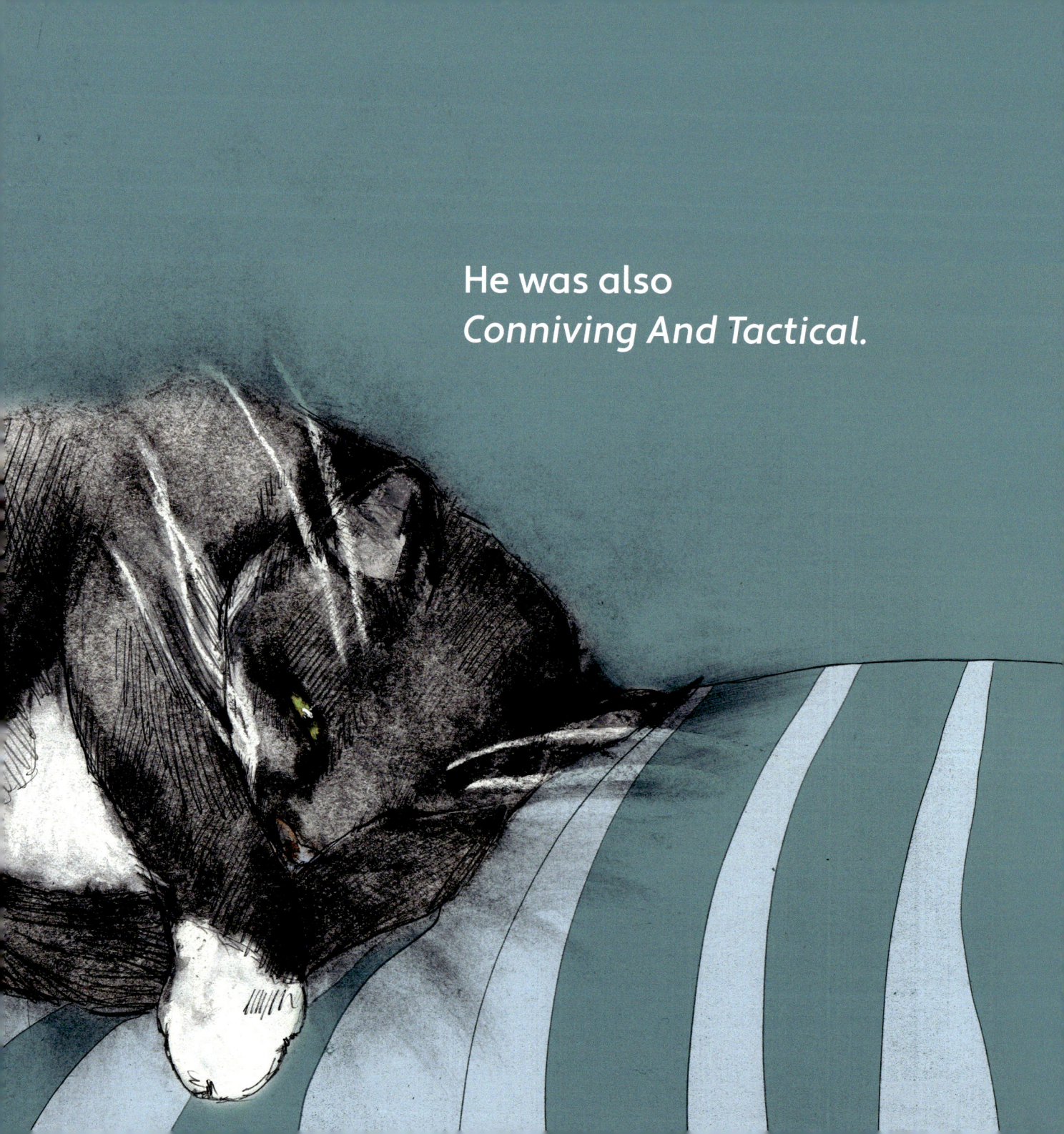

Pippin's favourite thing to do was to go to sleep.

But his second favourite thing to do was HUNTING ...

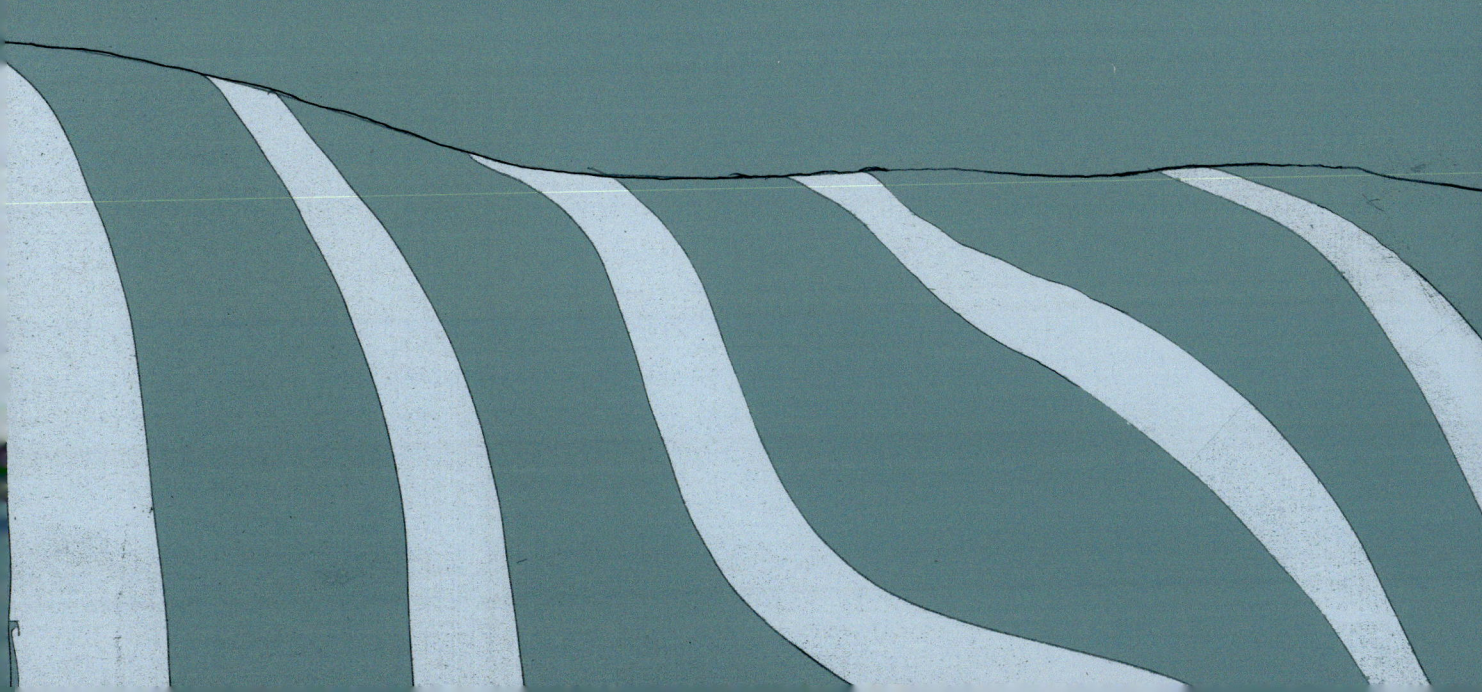

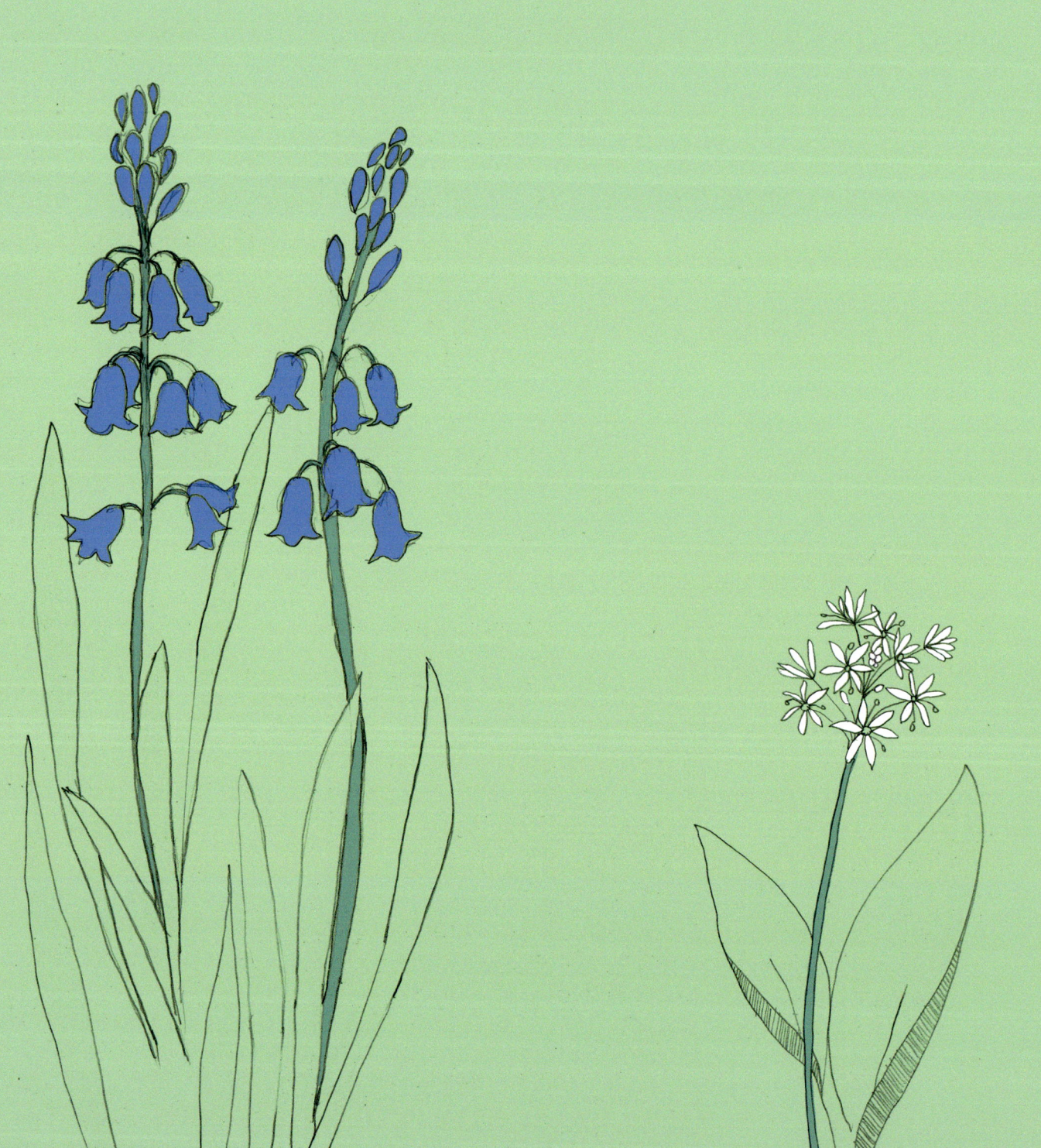

Pippin hunted shrews

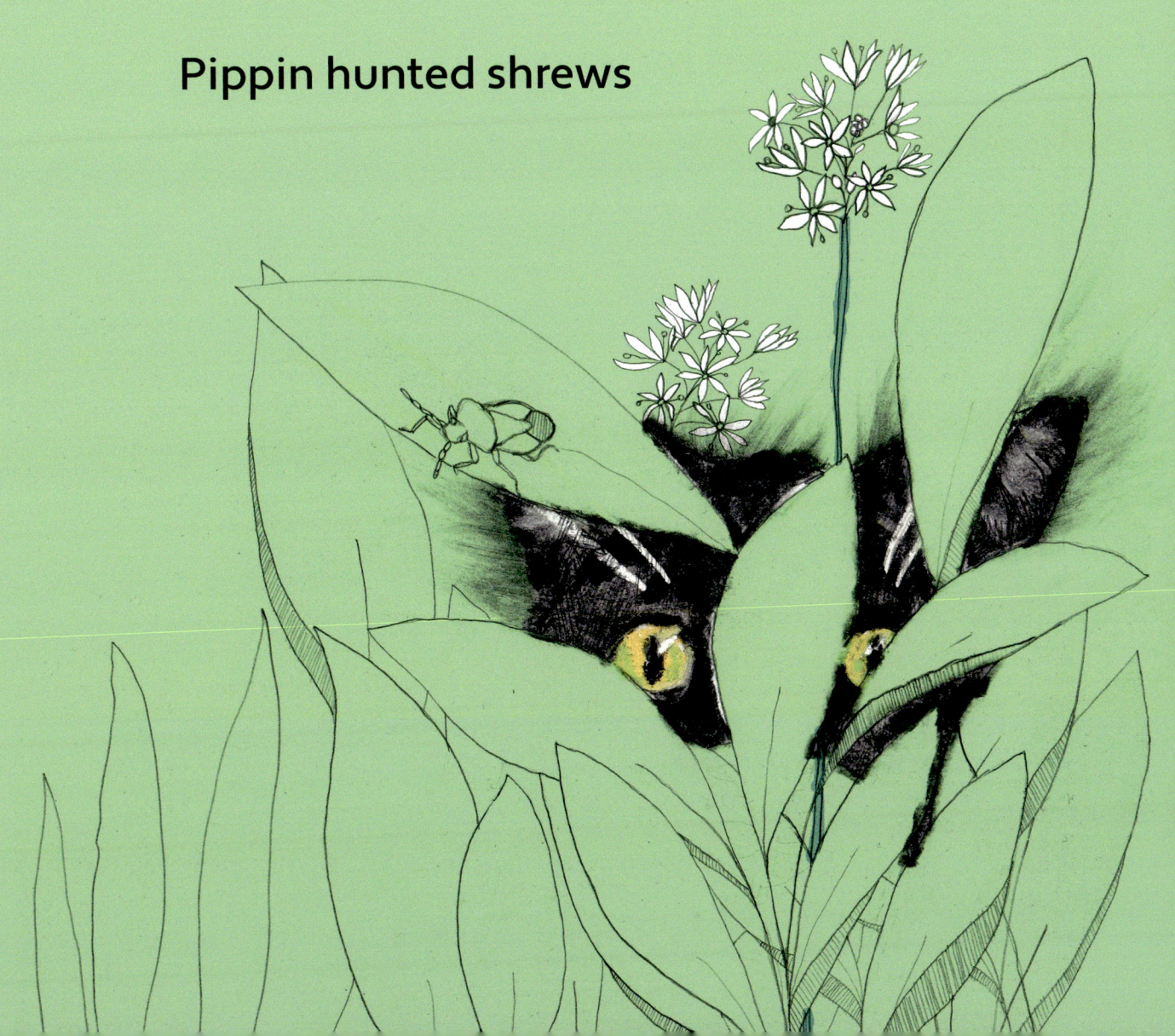

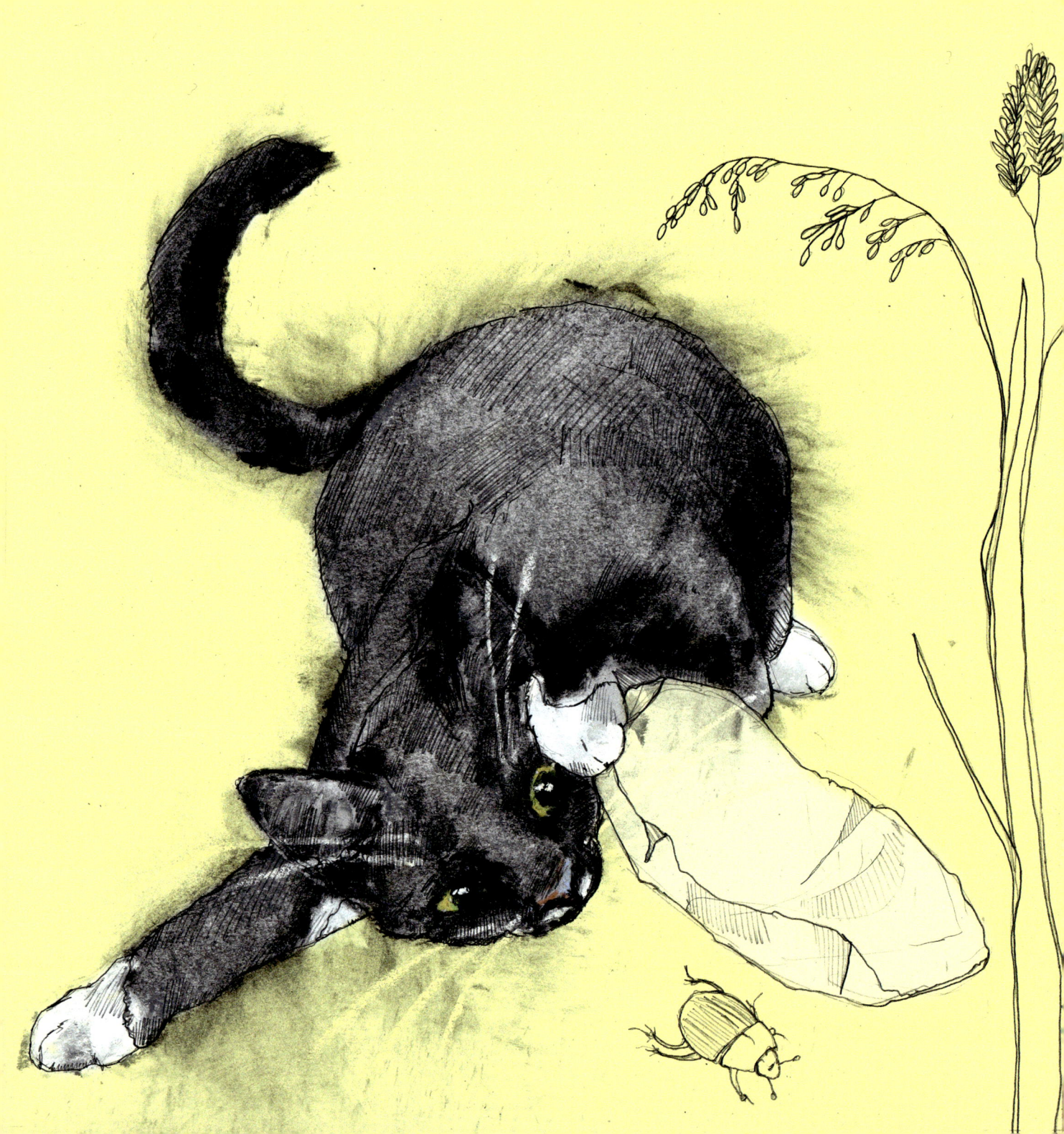

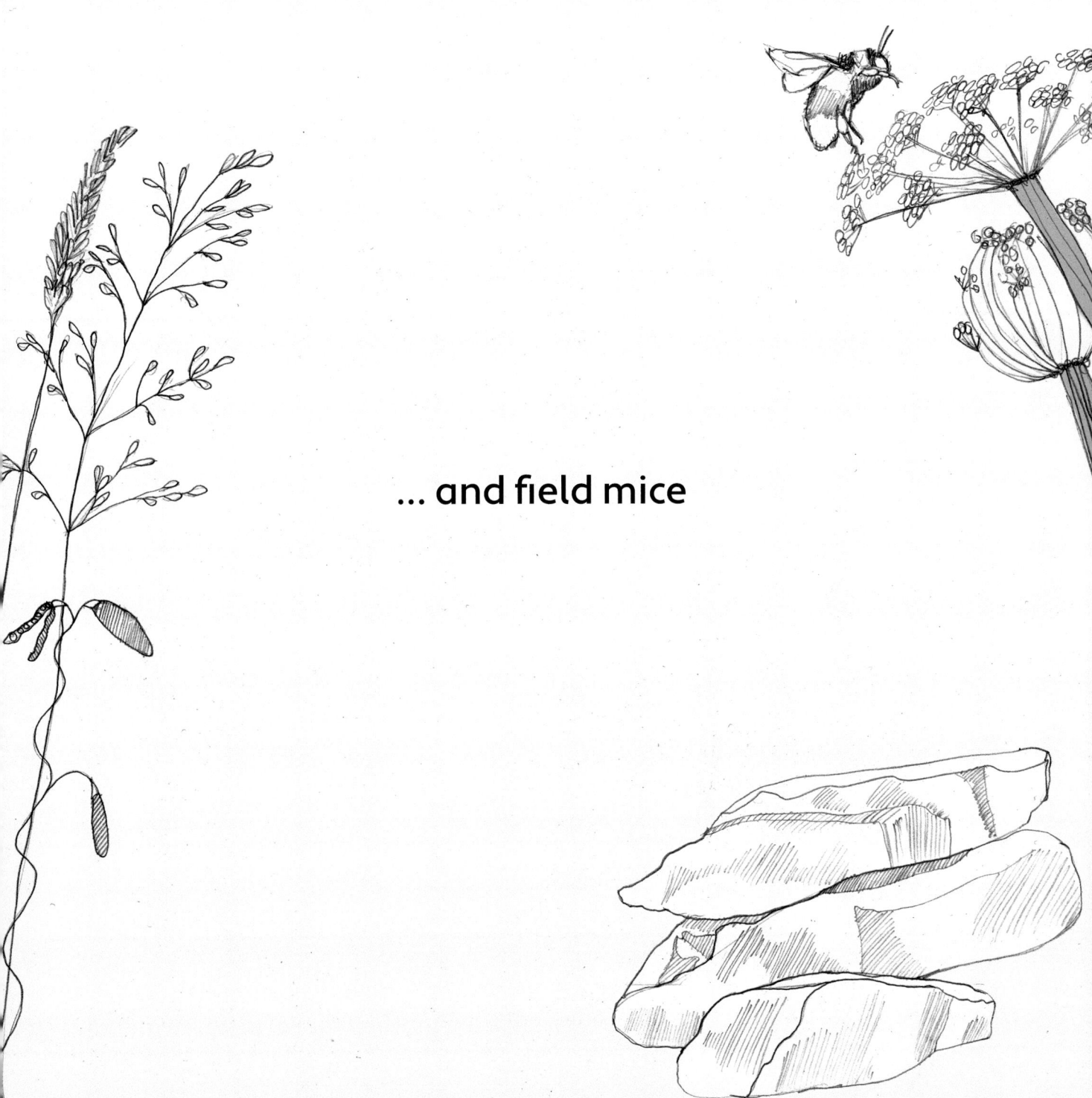
... and field mice

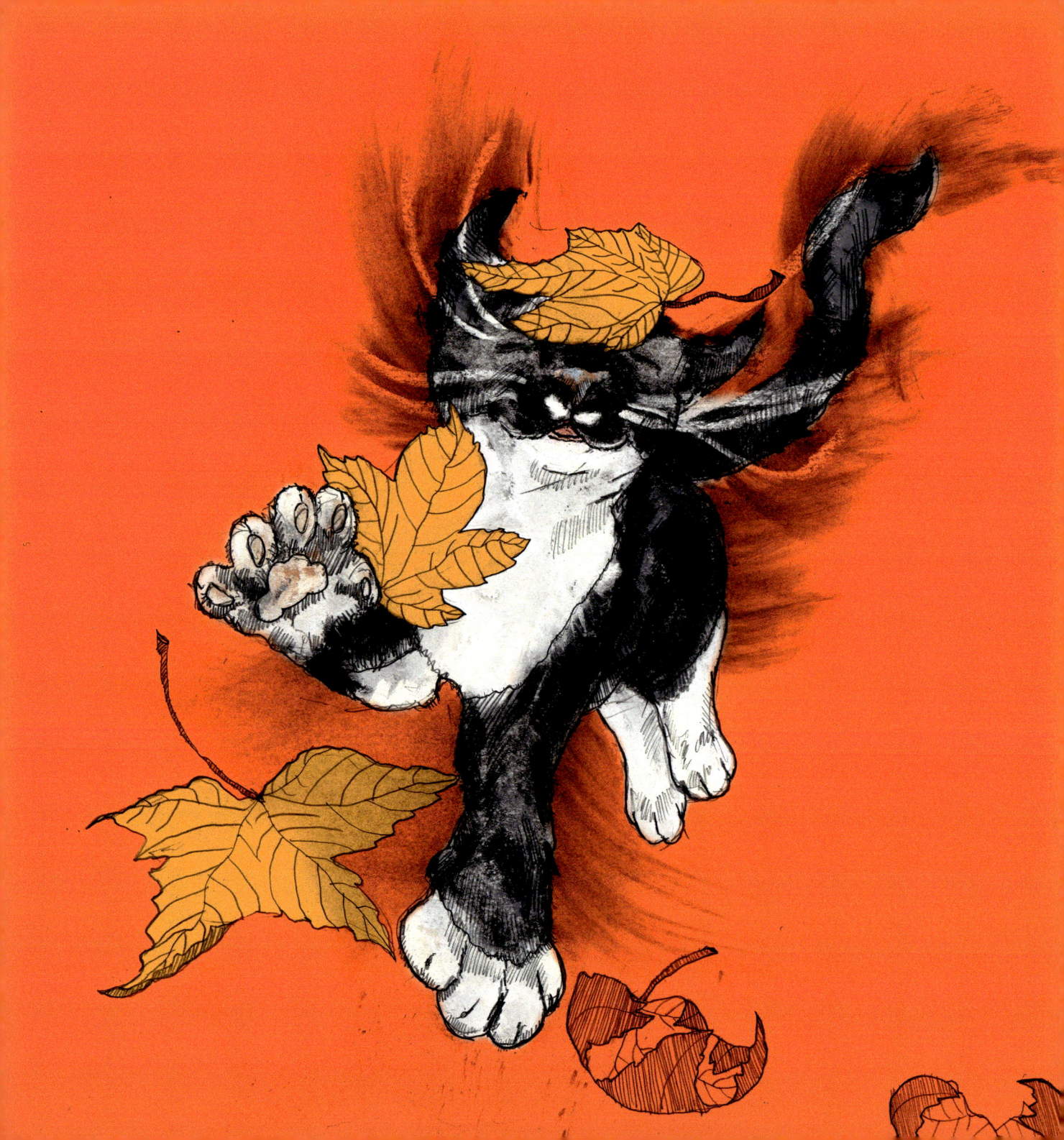

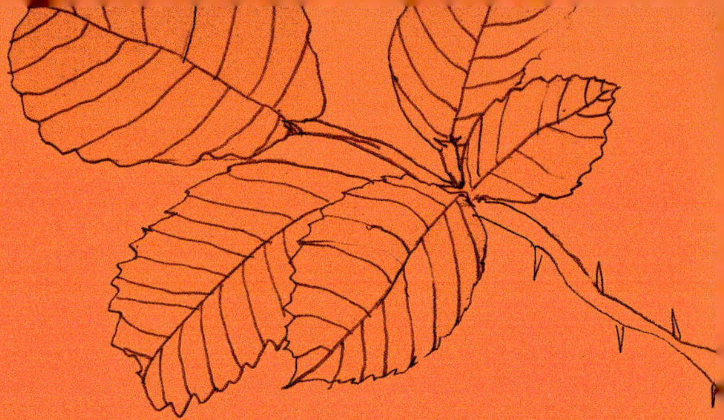

... and voles

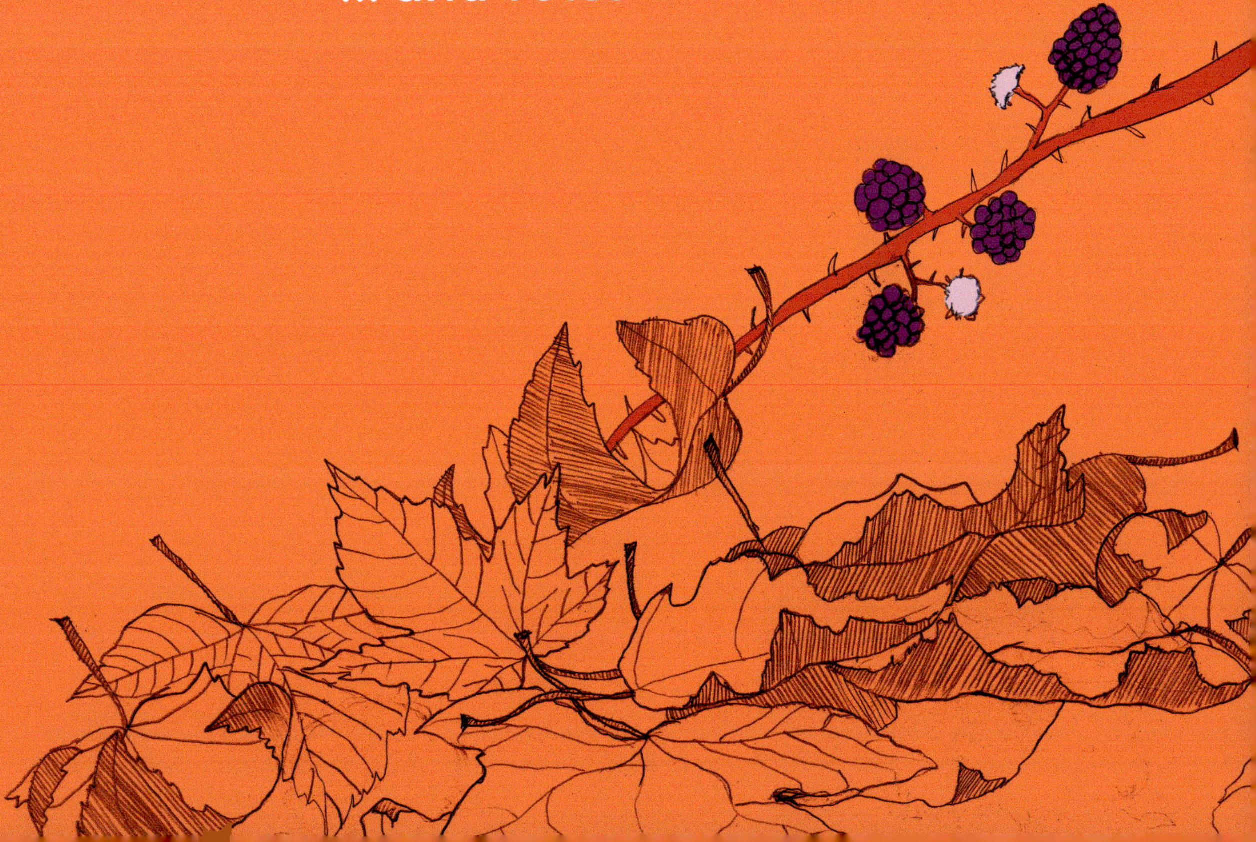

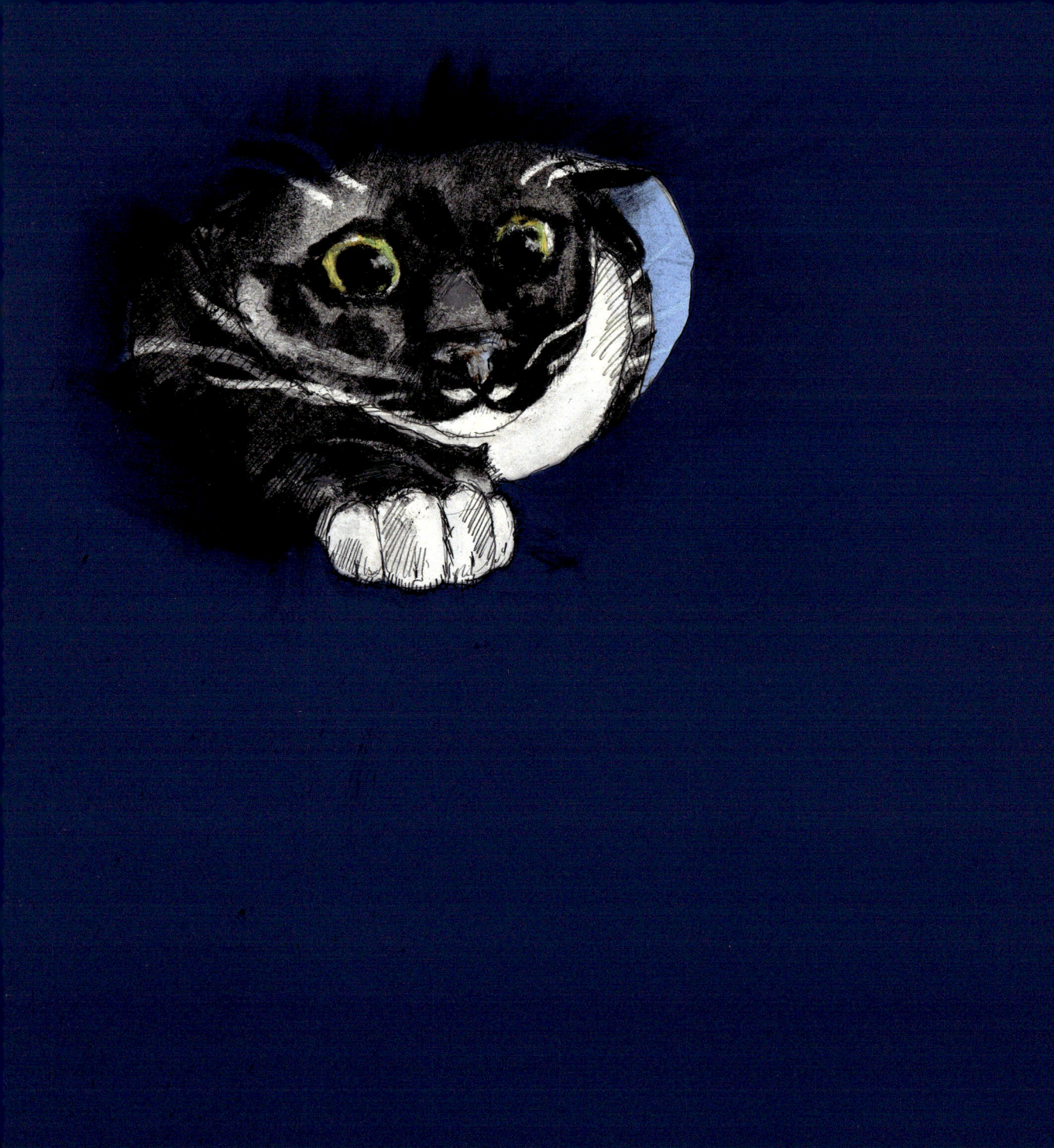

... and rabbits

... and he even hunted partridges.

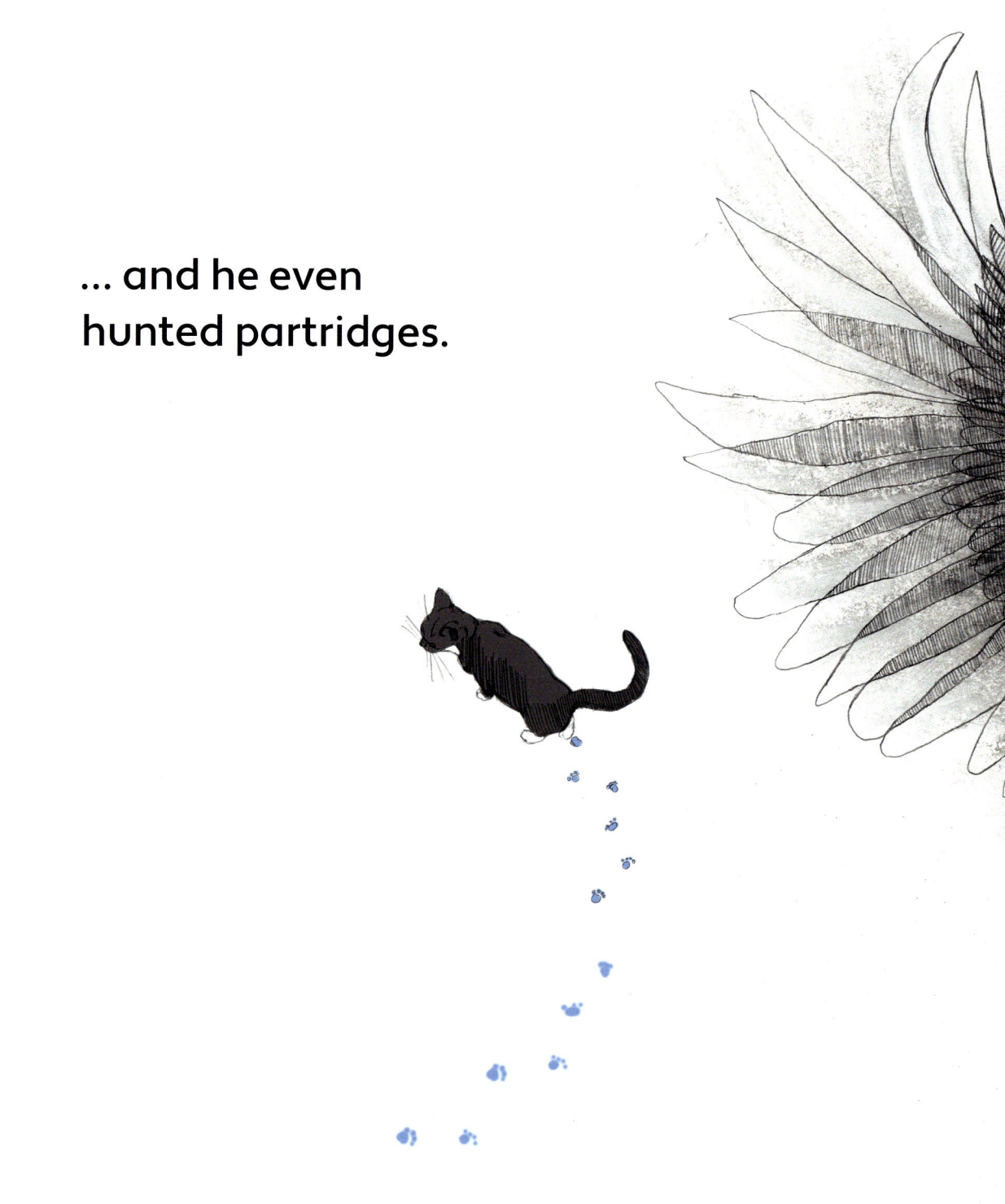

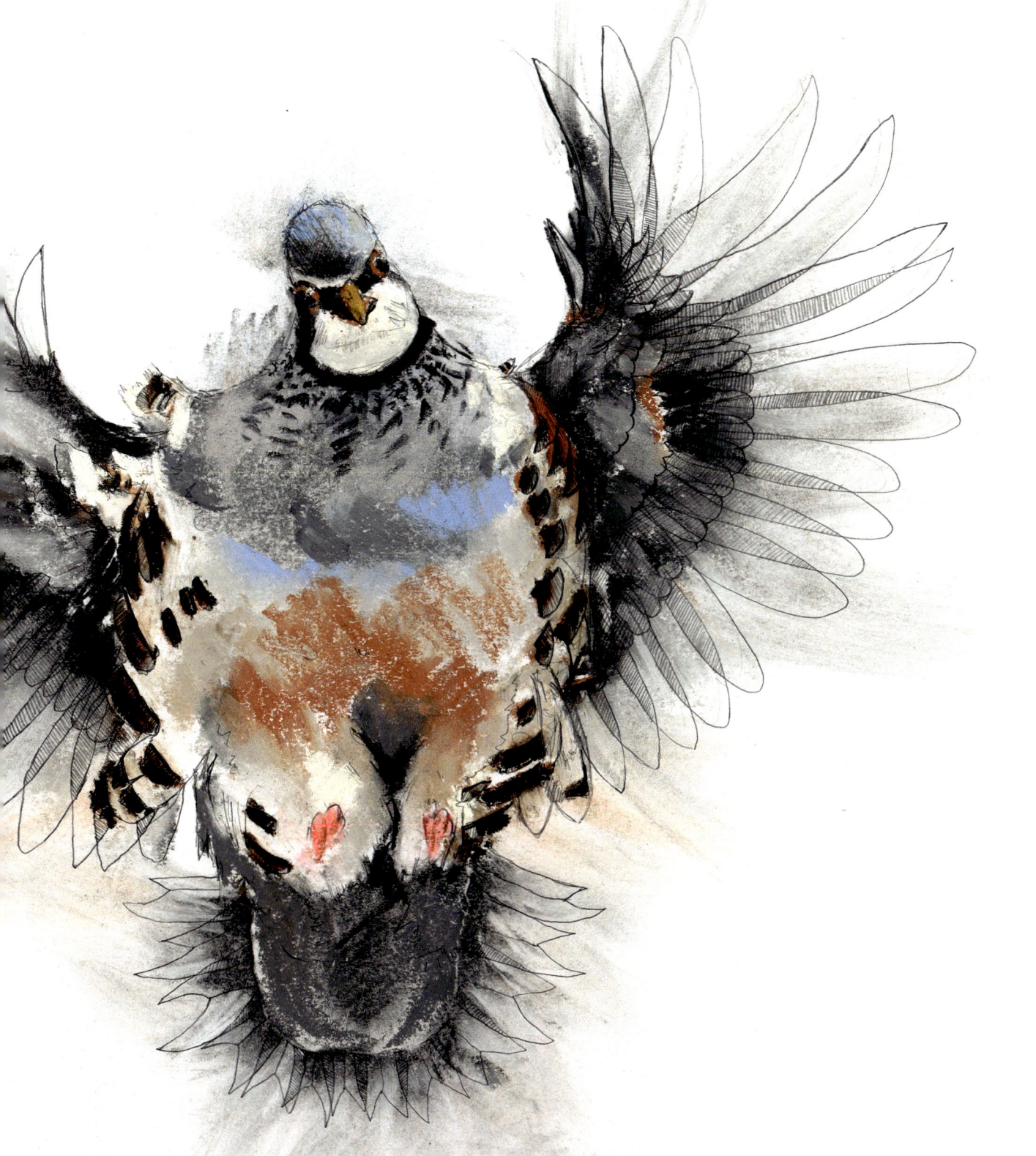

He brought all of his prey in through his cat flap and ate them on the bedroom floor – with NO TABLE MANNERS.

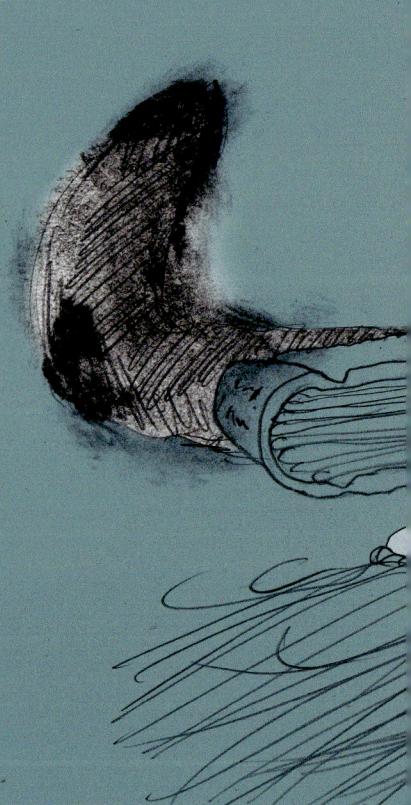

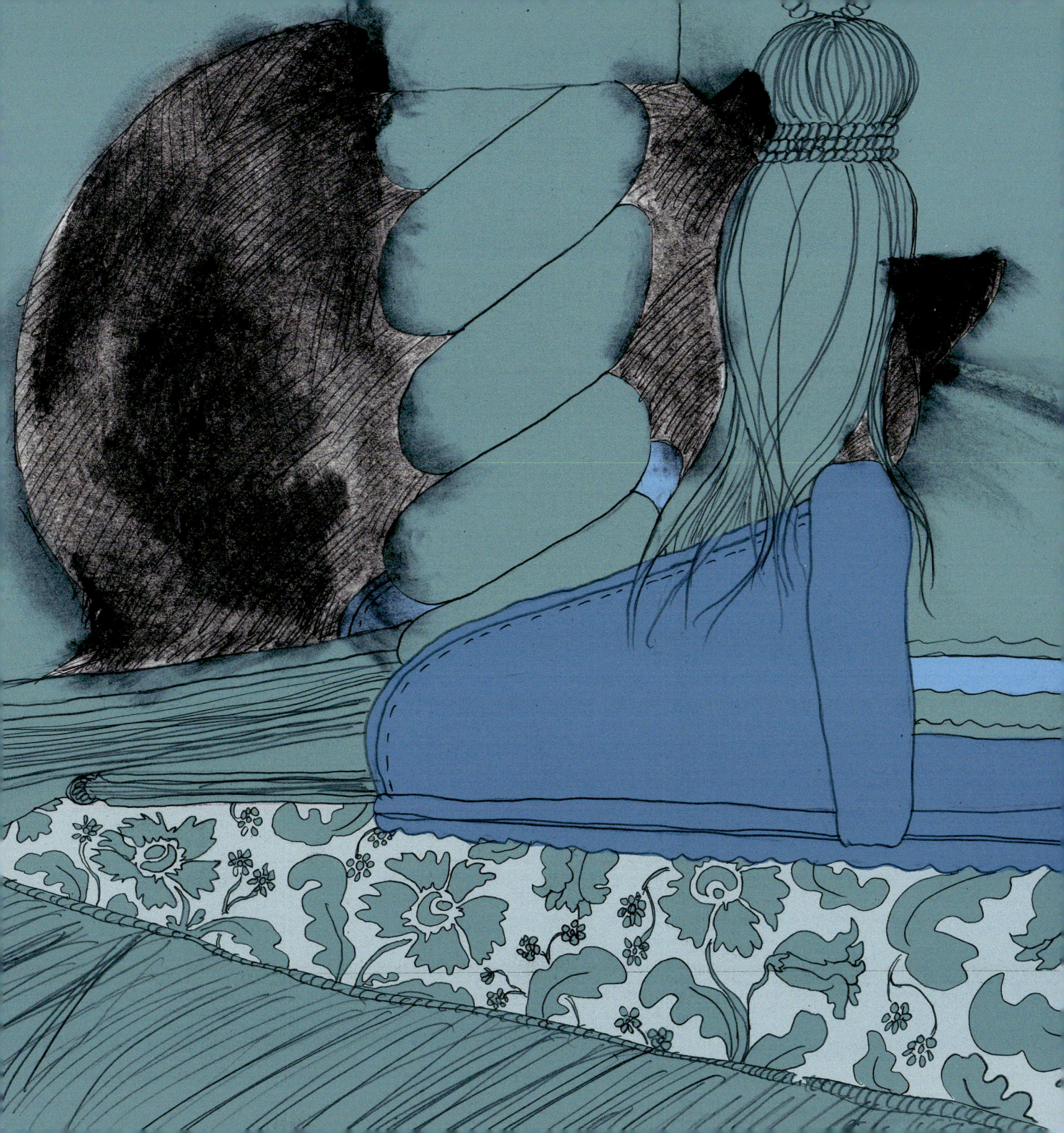

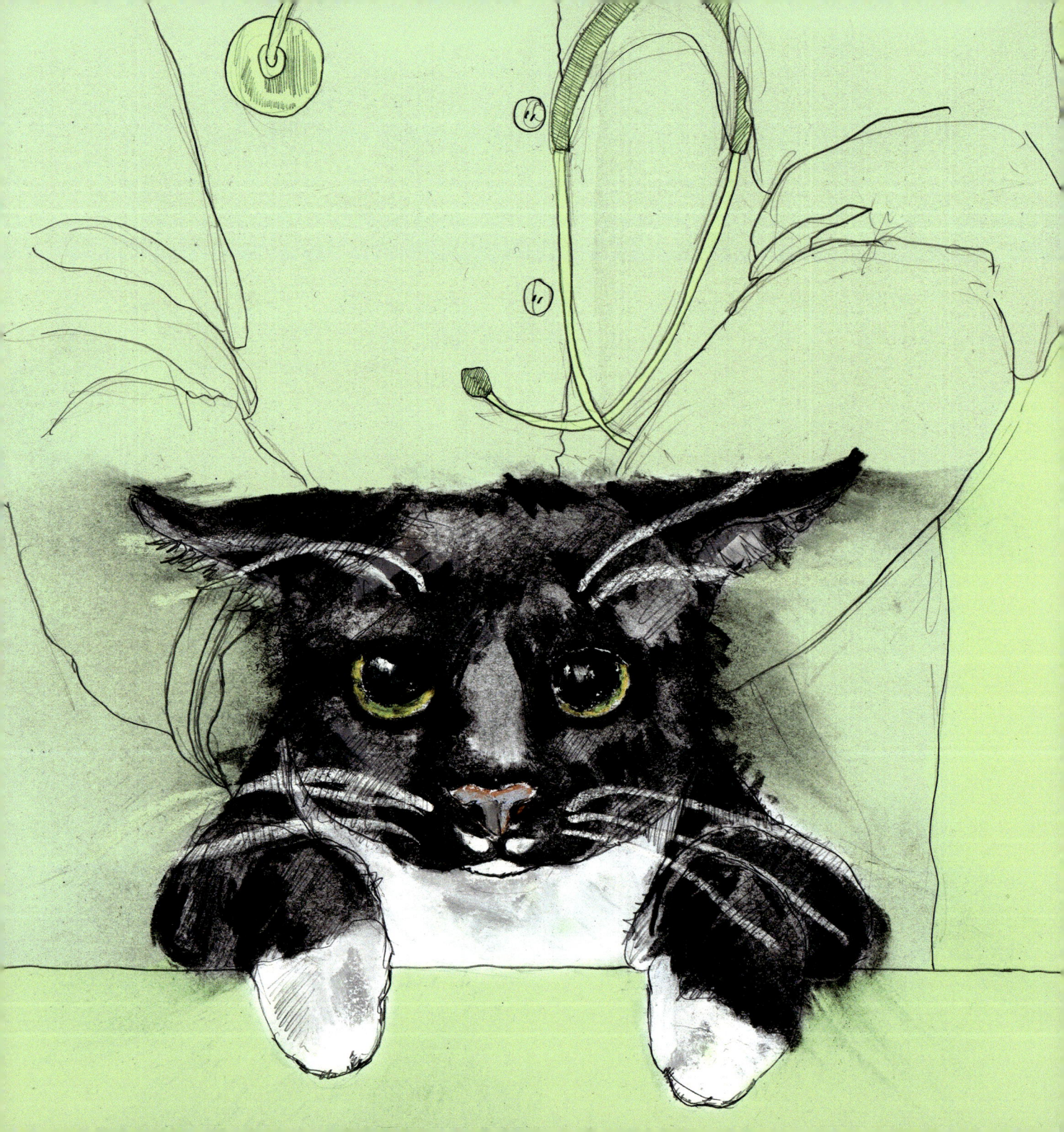

One day Pippin ate a bad vole
and he got sick.

So he was taken (in a cage – imagine it!)
to the vet and the vet gave him three sets
of medicine to take.

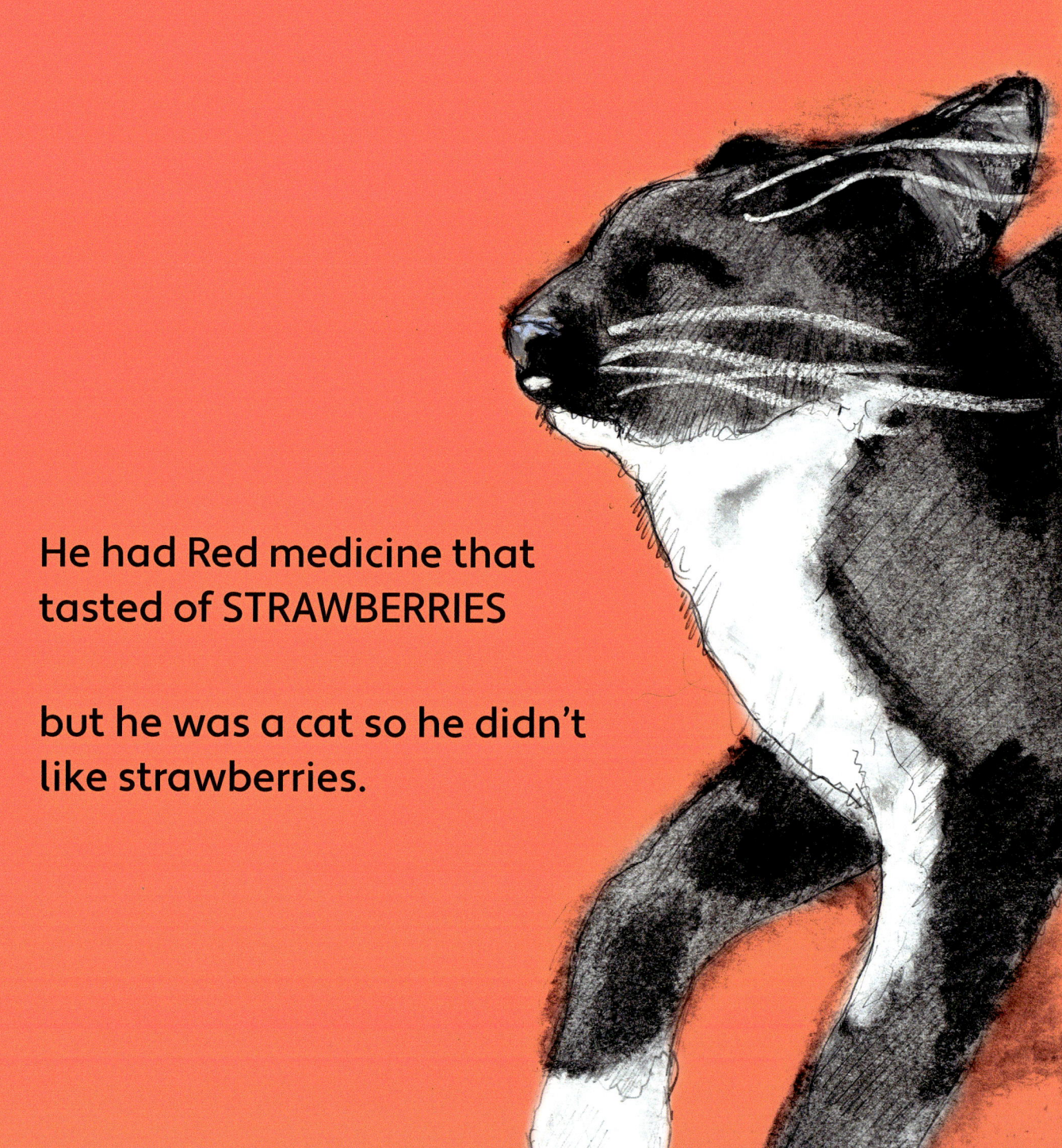

He had Red medicine that tasted of STRAWBERRIES

but he was a cat so he didn't like strawberries.

He had Yellow medicine that tasted of BANANAS

but he was a cat so he didn't like bananas.

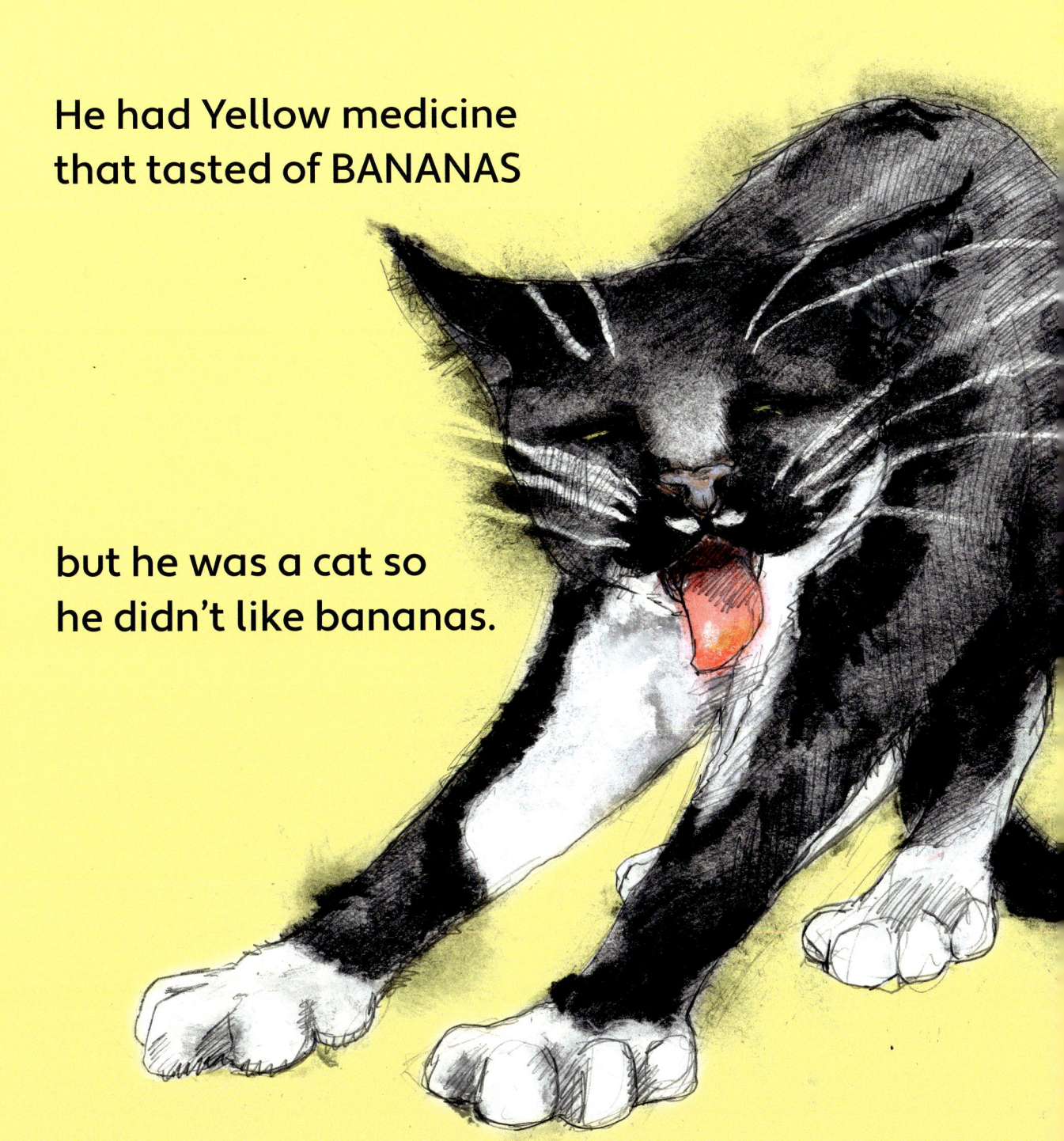

He had White medicine that tasted

DISGUSTING.

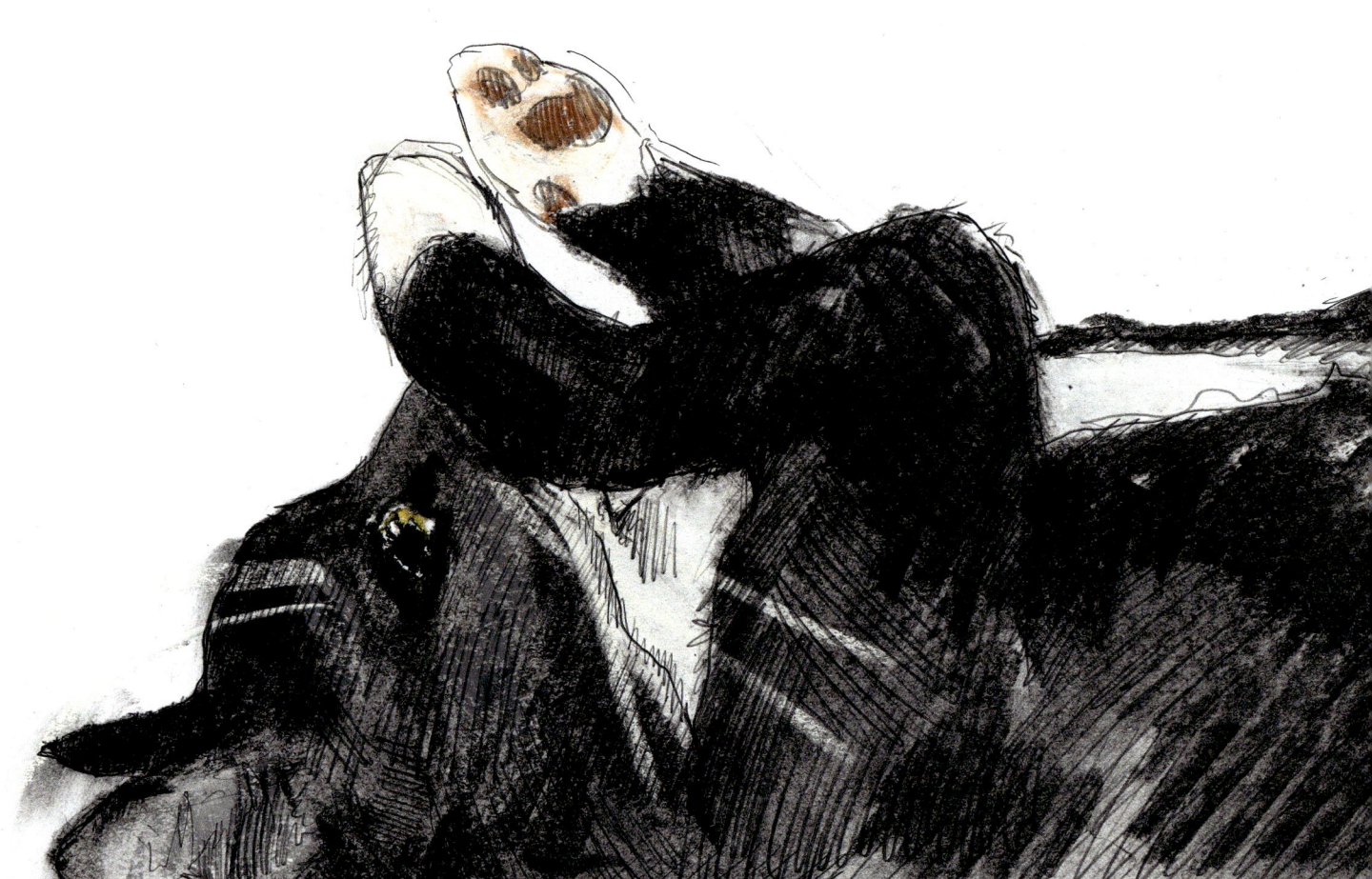

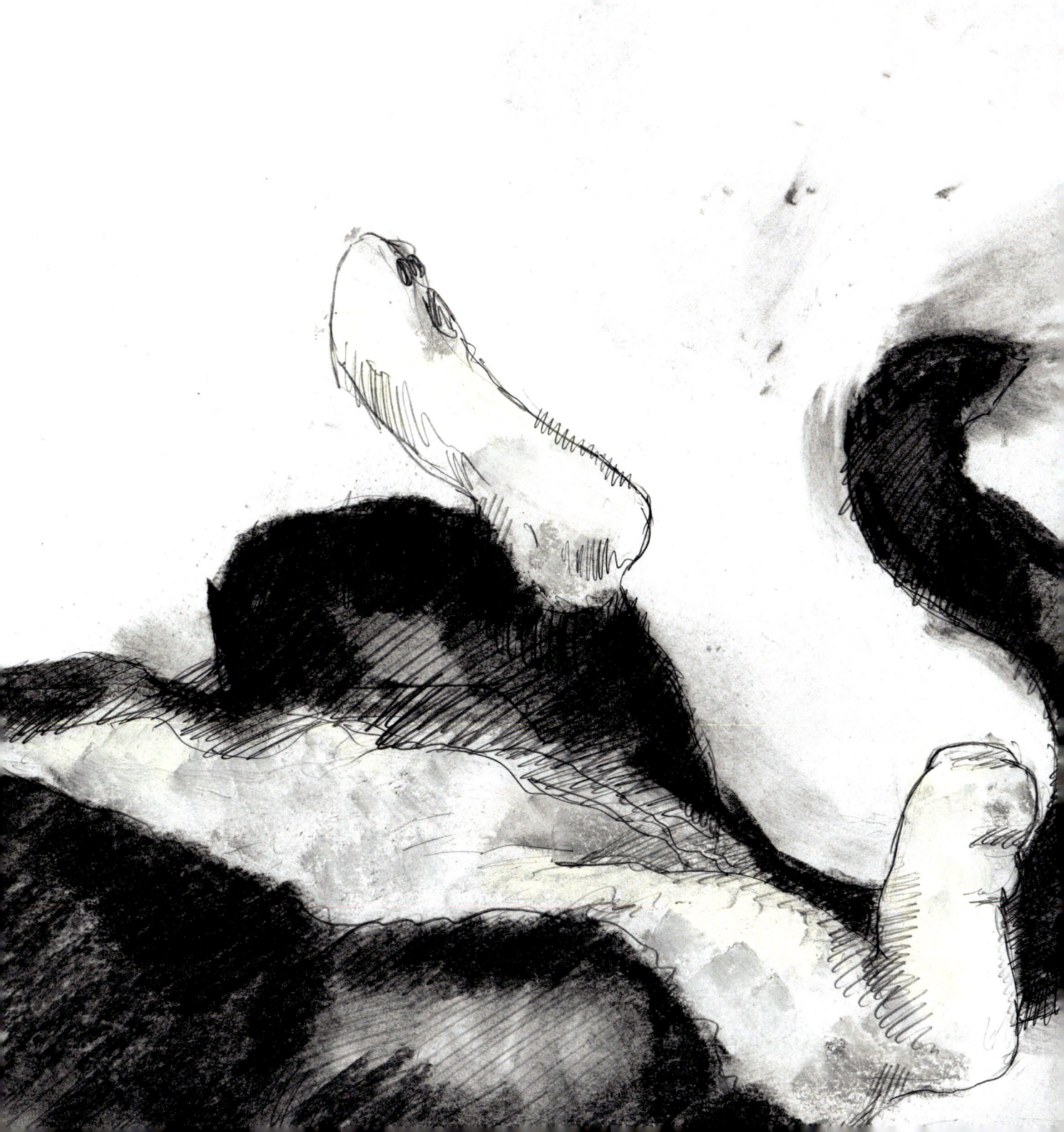

At this point Pippin became
Conniving And Tactical.

He hid behind the curtain.

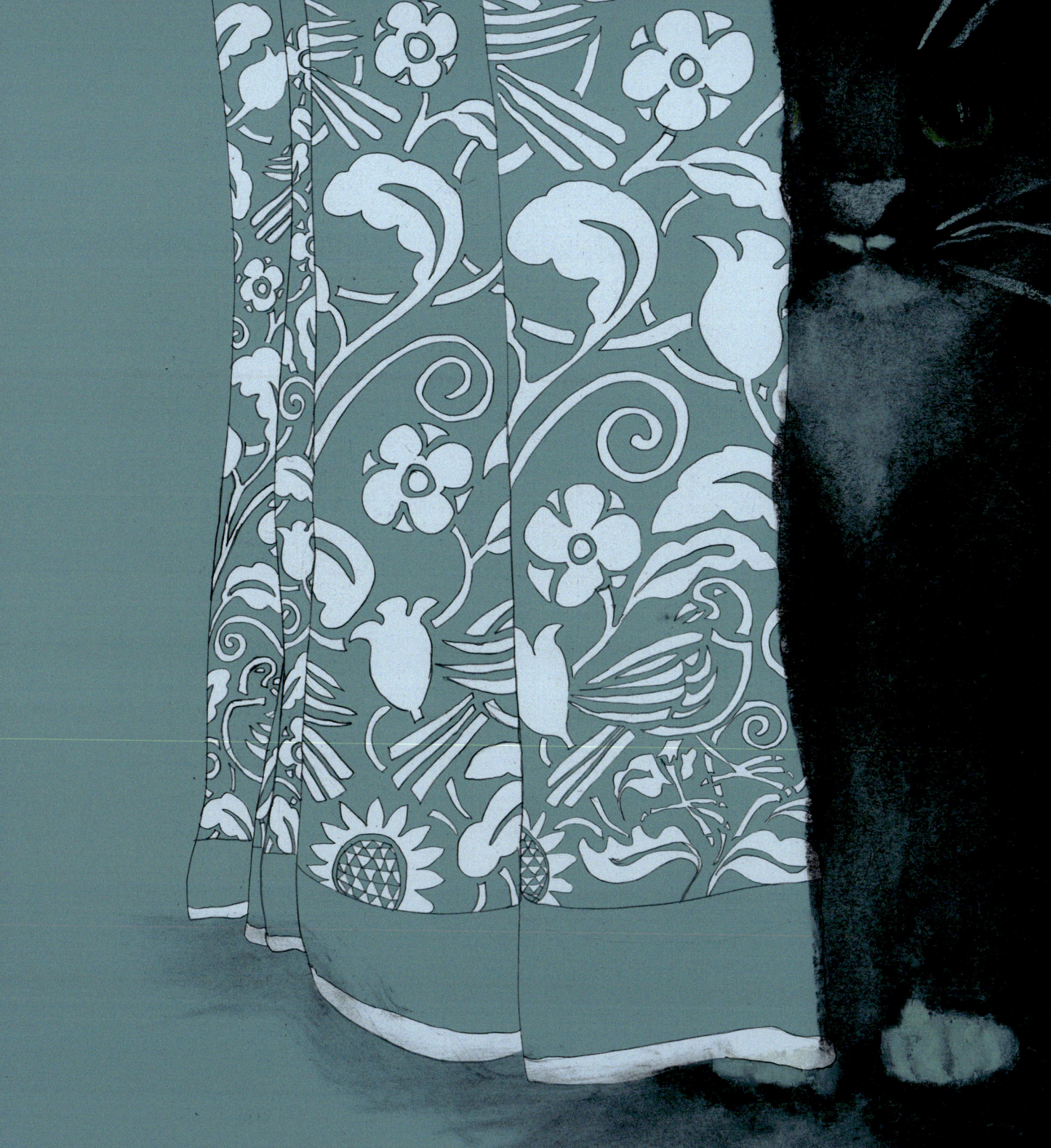

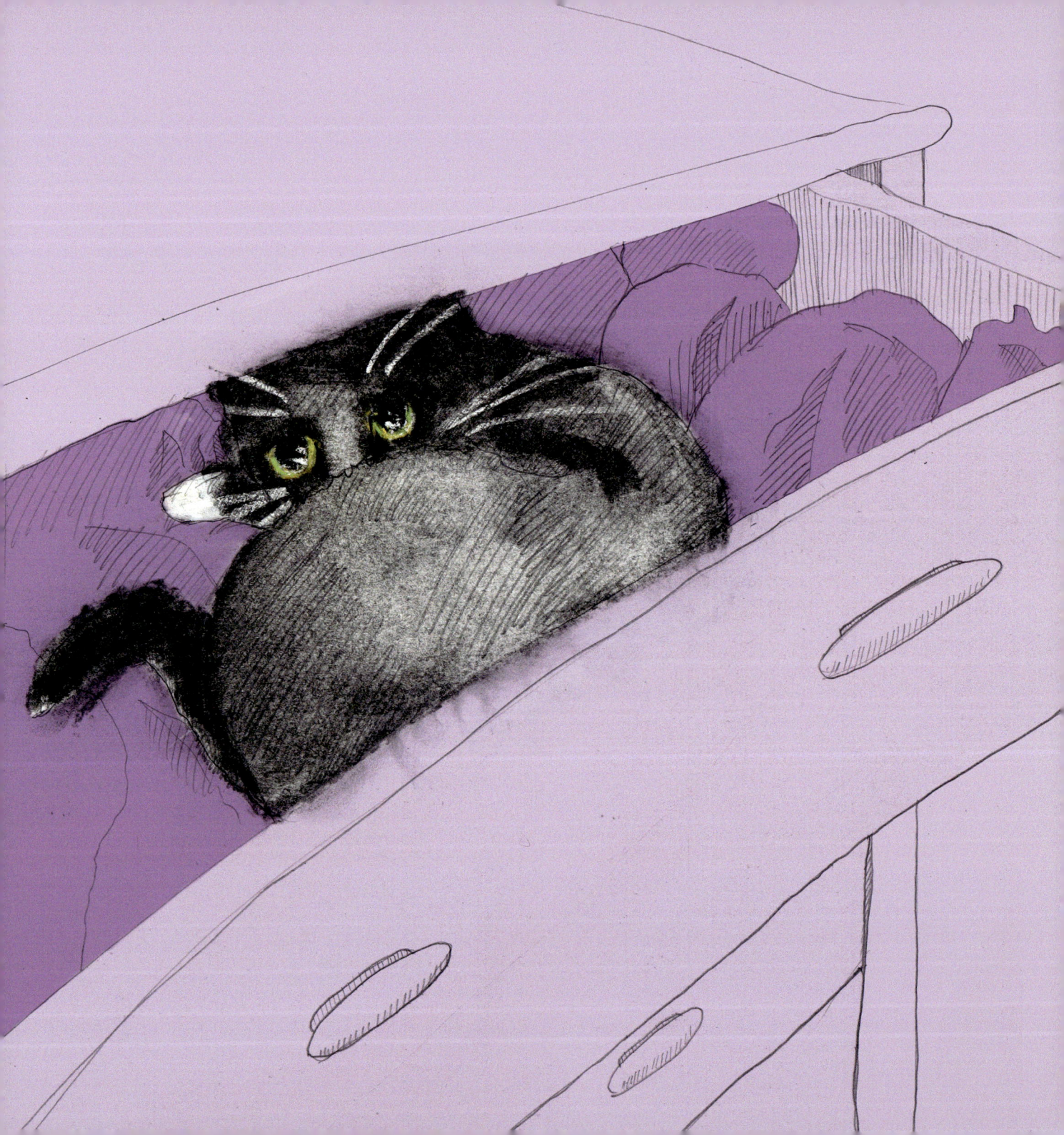

He hid in the drawer.

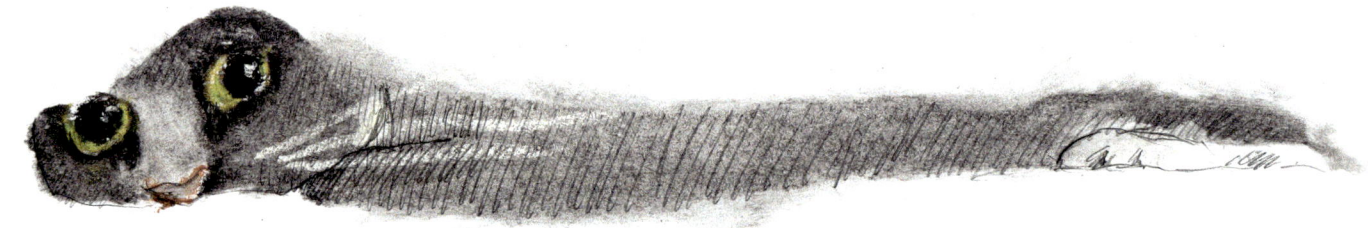

He learned how to open
the airing cupboard door

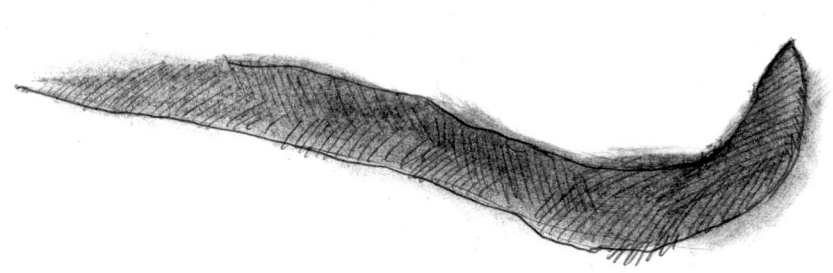

and he hid among
the clean sheets.

And when it wasn't raining he hid outside under the hedge.

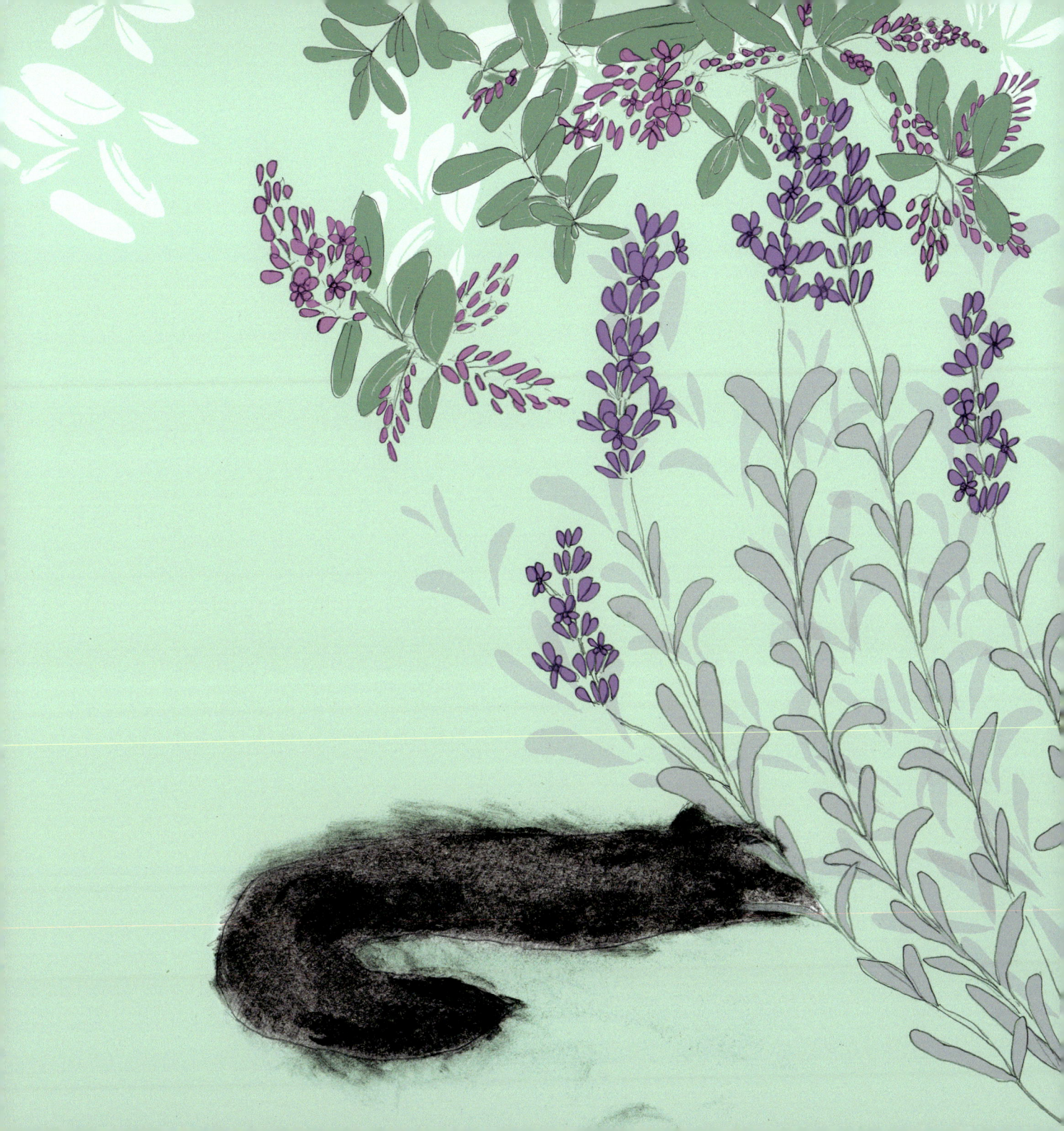

He was allowed all sorts of special treats: sour cream (yum), gravy (yum yum), and German Sausage (yum yum YUM).

But they didn't take away the taste of that horrid medicine.

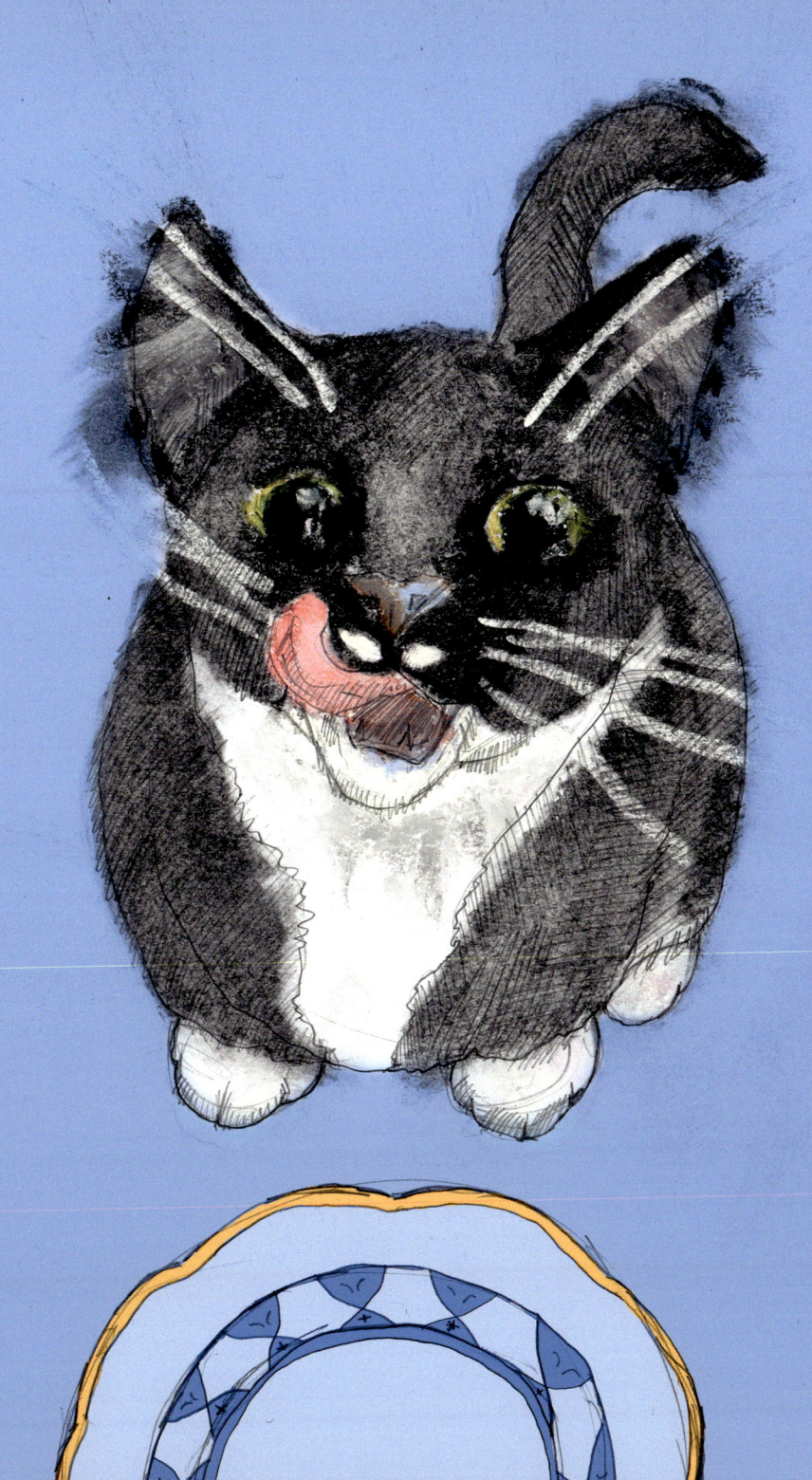

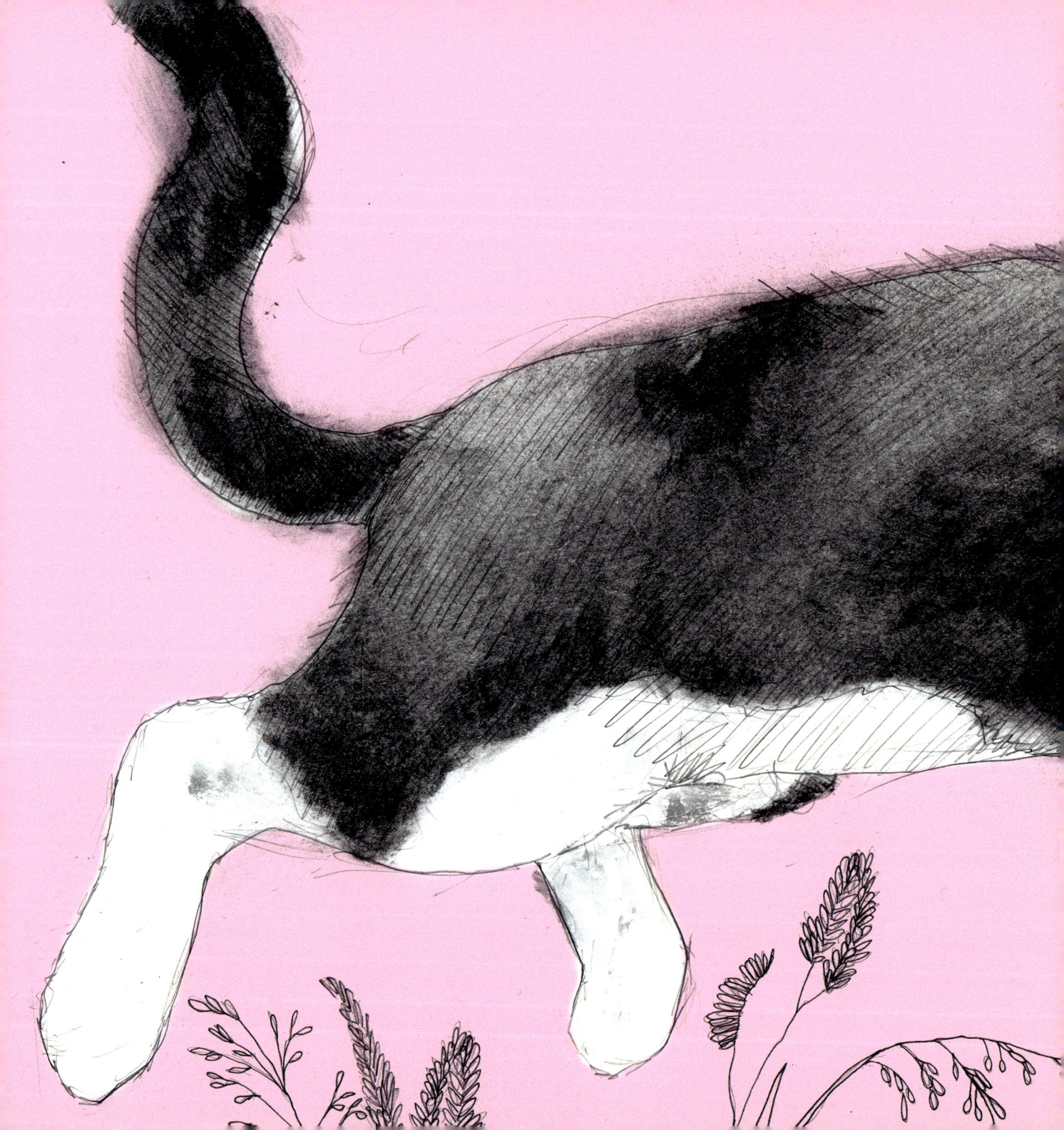

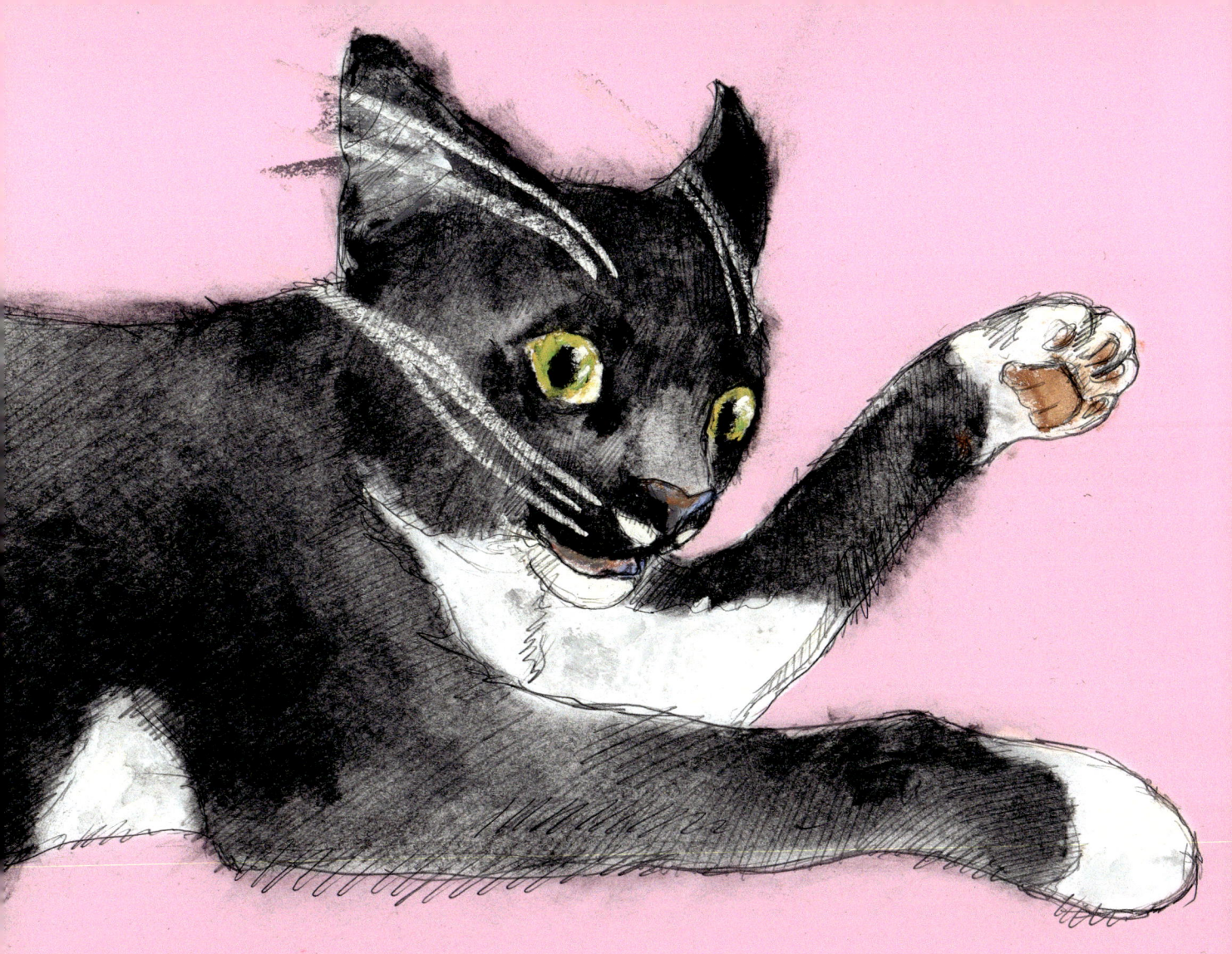

Eventually all the medicine was finished and Pippin felt Much Better.

And do you know what he did to celebrate?

He went out and caught himself a nice fat VOLE and he ate it on the bedroom floor with NO TABLE MANNERS.

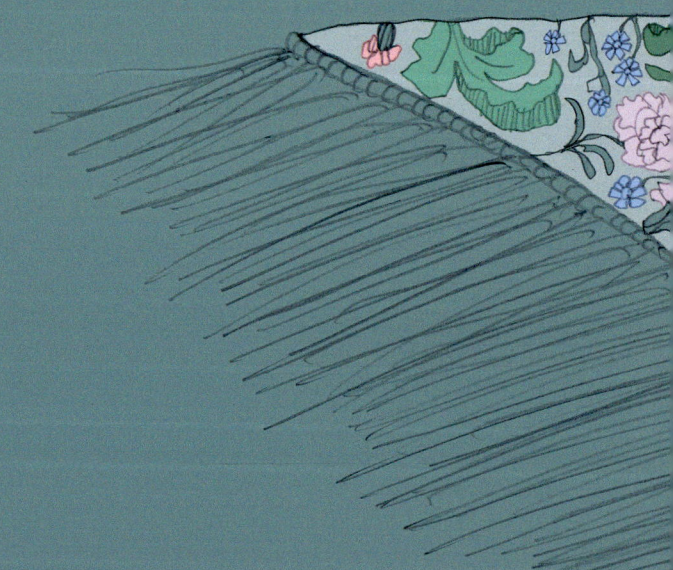

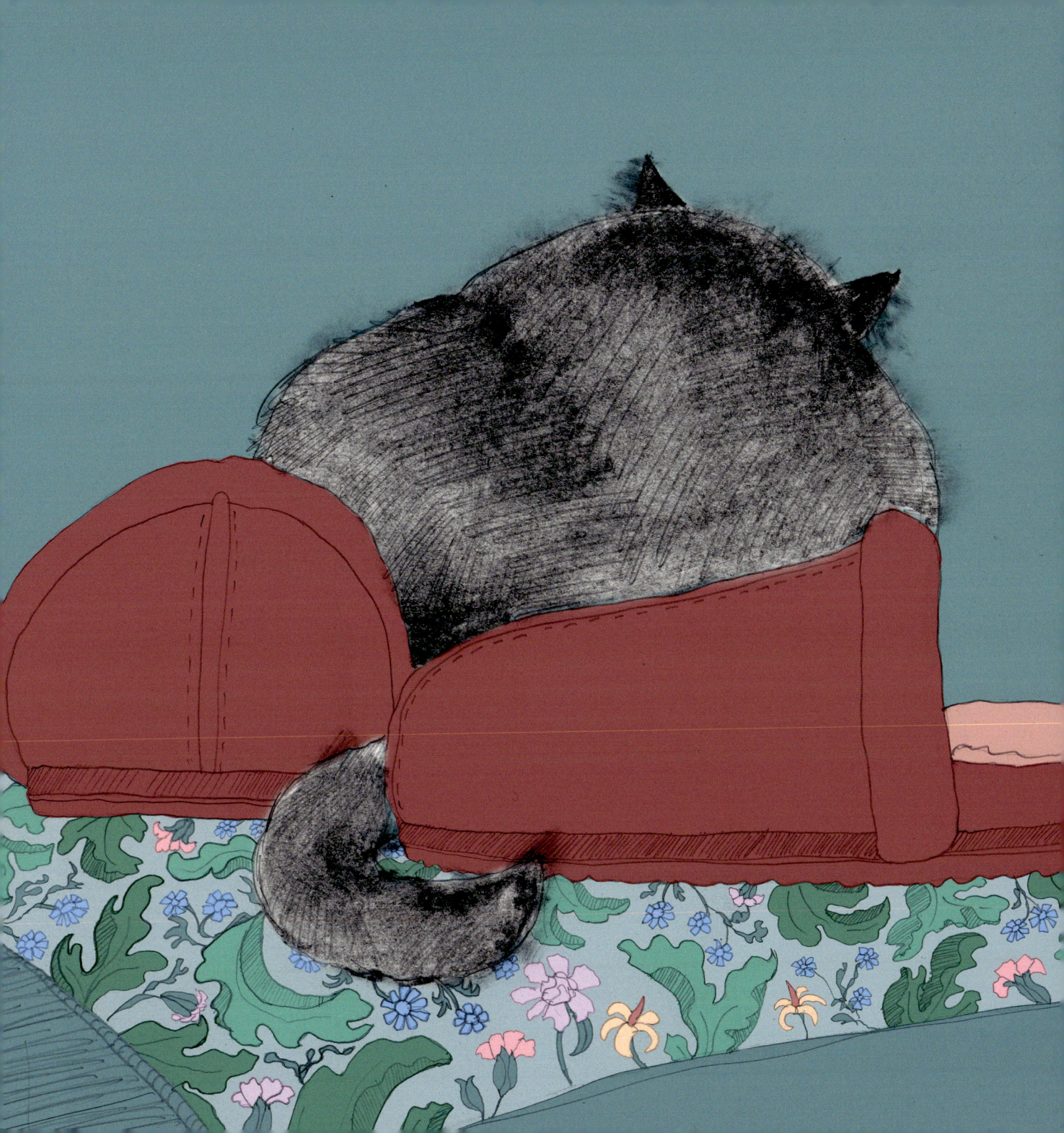

THE END

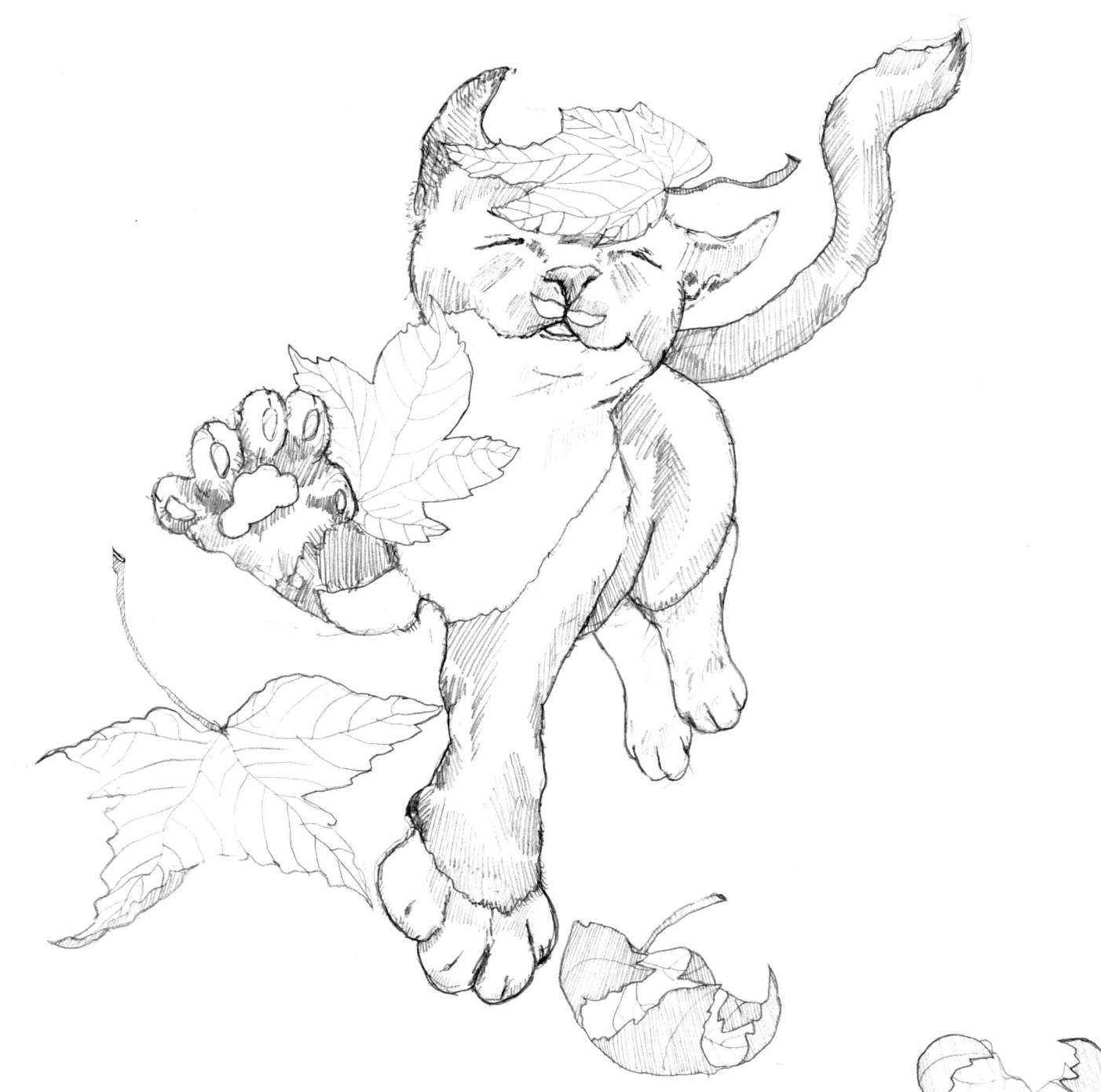

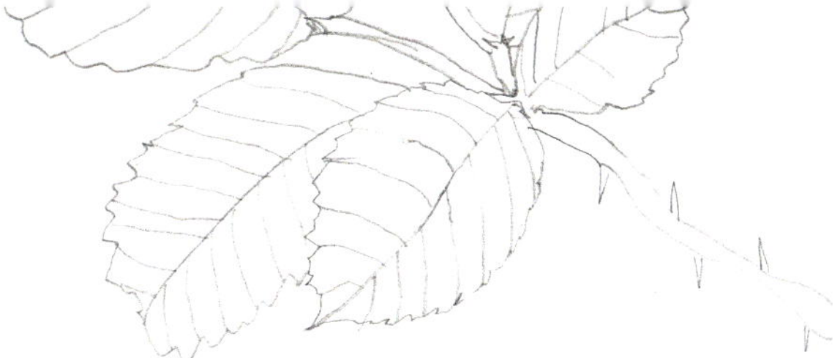

This is a true story. Pippin did indeed eat a 'bad vole' and he contracted a form of Tuberculosis from it, caused by *Mycobacterium microti*.

M. microti is found in Western Europe in the wild vole population, and also apparently in llamas, but I don't think Pippin ever ate a llama. Pippin became the western-most case of *M.microti* ever seen in a domestic cat in Europe, which made the vets very excited.

For his treatment he was prescribed triple therapy with Rifamycin, Erythromycin and Veraflox (pradofloxacin) which in the end he took for four months.

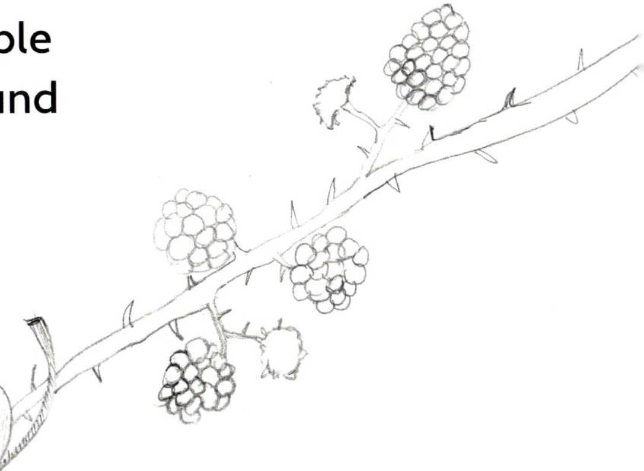

Thankfully, the treatment worked and he soon felt Much Better.

Penny

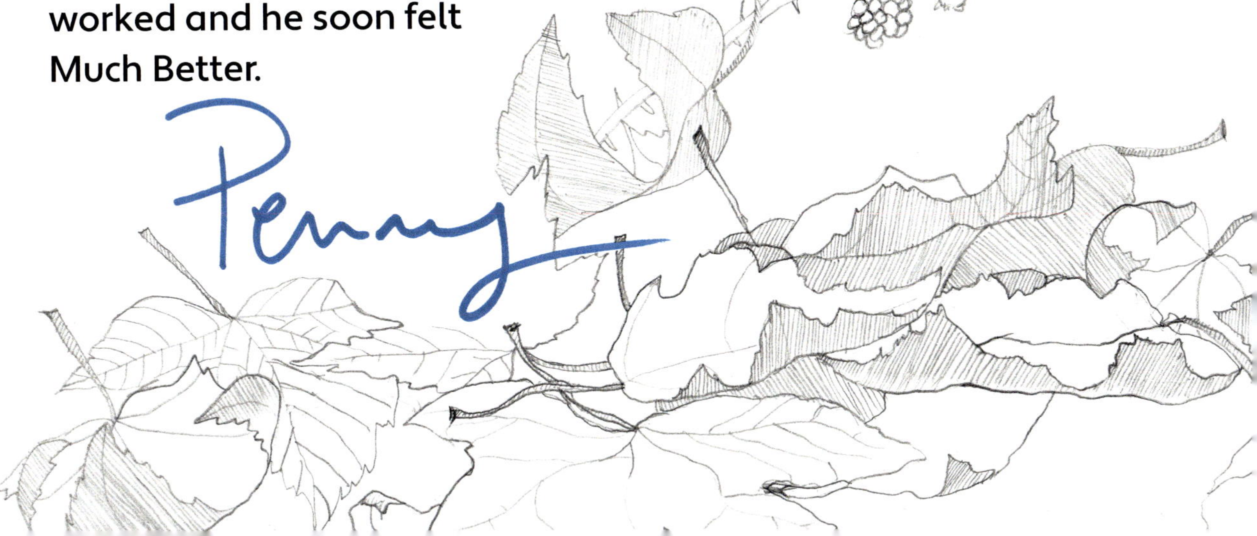